ALLERGIES AND INFECTIOUS DISEASES

JOURNEY THROUGH THE WORLD OF MALARIA

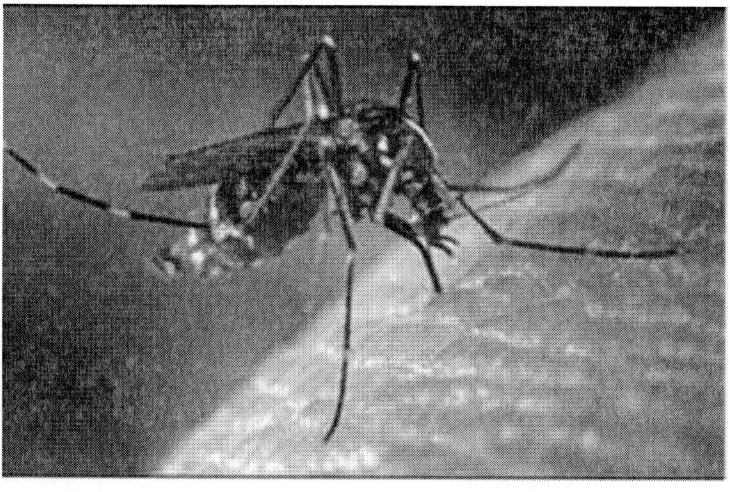

ALLERGIES AND INFECTIOUS DISEASES

Additional books in this series can be found on Nova's website under the Series tab.

Additional e-books in this series can be found on Nova's website under the e-book tab.

ALLERGIES AND INFECTIOUS DISEASES

JOURNEY THROUGH THE WORLD OF MALARIA

ABUBAKAR YARO (KHALIFA)
FOUNDER & CEO
AFRICA HEALTH RESEARCH ORGANIZATION

NOVA BIOMEDICAL

New York

For permission to use material from this book please contact us:
Telephone 631-231-7269; Fax 631-231-8175
Web Site: http://www.novapublishers.com

Additional color graphics may be available in the e-book version of this book.

Library of Congress Cataloging-in-Publication Data

ISBN: 978-1-62948-636-9

Library of Congress Control Number: 2014931904

Published by Nova Science Publishers, Inc. † New York

To

Bill & Melinda Gates

My Children

My mum, Amina Ahmed

My dad, Abdullah Yaro

My beloved late aunt, Madame Izatu

Contents

Preface

"Malaria disaster in Africa" was the heading of a letter by Kevin Marsh to *Lancet* in September 1998. A disaster, he stated, which is not just on its way but already happening. This strong warning was prompted as a result of a report by Trape et al. on the changing pattern of mortality in three areas of Senegal over an 11-year period in regions which represented three different transmission levels. There have been tremendous developments in the area of malarialogy. Despite all the successes that have been achieved, malaria remains one of the world's most serious public health issues with an estimated 1.5 to 2.7 million or more deaths annually. The cases are concentrated among pregnant women and children.

Significantly more people are dying from malaria today than 30 years ago. Drug resistance is posing even more challenges than ever with the world running against time to either develop new antimalarial agents or to optimize the existing agents. A malaria vaccine remains elusive. Although there has been some interesting data made available, the scientific barrier has yet to be broken. Human apathy towards malaria control is derailing the global effort. Some of these factors will be reviewed in this book. The book begins with a critical analysis of the history and classification of malaria. In Chapter 1, the malaria parasite and its life cycle are reviewed. The *Plasmodium* genome and metabolism is briefly analyzed. In Chapter 2, recent advances in the epidemiology of malaria are examined. This ranges from the polymerase chain reaction to current situations and distribution and mortality patterns. Chapter 3 looks at the pathogenesis of the infection. Subtopics include the parasite and the immune system, HLA system and malaria, measuring virulence and clinical manifestation. Some of the complications associated with malaria infection are reviewed in detail. In Chapter 4, an update on malaria treatments and drug resistance is analyzed. This includes an overview of the main classes of antimalarial drugs. The available regimen, ACT is reviewed in detail. The mechanism of drug resistance is also discussed. Control strategies are covered in Chapter 5. Some of the issues in this chapter include the economic and social burden of malaria and various recommended control strategies with vaccinations reviewed in detail.

I hope this book will help stimulate debate and discussion on malaria which in the end will help humanity to deal with this emerging public health concern.

Acknowledgements

My gratitude goes to my Creator for His Mercies without which I couldn't have achieved so much. If I am to name somebody as co-author of this book, it would be my late father, Alhaji Abdullah Yaro who not only instilled in me the spirit of hard work but also its simplicity. Dad, thank you. My next thanks go to my mum, Amina Ahmed who once challenged me to fight hard to become a scientist. That challenge kept me focused during the most difficult part of my life. Mum, thanks a million times. What I am today symbolizes the energy expended by my teachers, lecturers, and many others. They are too many to be mentioned but for each one of you out there thanks for teaching me great things. My children gave me the strength of love which I missed most. This gave me the hope and energy to go all out. Thanks to my kids! To my wives, thanks for being the bed of comfort who provided me with shoulders to cry on when things were really bad and all my friends deserted me.

Thanks to all of the members of the Africa Health Research Organization, who supported me through thick and thin. Today we are almost there. Thanks for your belief in me. To all the authors of the studies used in putting together this book, I want to thank you for the wonderful work you've given to the world. Without such efforts, I couldn't have written this book. Special mention must also be made of the following organizations and individuals who gave me the permission to use their data: Center for Disease Control (CDC, USA), Dr. Louis Miller (NIH, USA), Dr. Kakkilaya (India) and Dr Ananias A. Escalante (Arizona State University, USA). I also want to thank Mr. Rich Van Lue of Author House for the encouragement he gave me while working rather reluctantly on this book. Had he not persisted in putting pressure on me, this book would not have seen the light of day.

To Nova Science Publishers, especially Professor Michael Popejoy, thanks for giving me the opportunity to fulfill a childhood ambition of writing books for humanity.

Cover page image: Mosquito biting a victim (Credit: CDC)

Chapter I

Introduction: History and Classification

Historical Perspective

Malaria has been with humanity for over 5,000 years. The term malaria originated from a Medieval Italian word "mala aria" which means "bad air". The disease was initially called "ague" or "marsh fever" because it was associated with swamps and marshland. This section will review the historical path of malaria chronicling the important events that shaped the field of malaria medicine. However, this is not a definitive account as some historical trends may have been missed.

In 1880, a French army doctor Charles Louis Alphonse Laveran working in a military hospital in Constantine Algeria first observed the parasite in the red blood cells of individuals suffering from malaria. He then proposed that malaria is caused by the parasite. In 1907, he was awarded the Nobel Peace Prize in Medicine & Physiology for his work. Four doctors had previously worked extensively on the disease including: F.C. Maillot who worked in North Africa and successfully developed quinine therapy; Leon Colin who was responsible for several epidemiological studies and Achille Kelsch and P.J. Keiner who undertook a pathological research, with Kelsch focusing on the malarial black pigment. In 1847, the German pathologist Heinrich Meckel first described the black pigment while in 1858 another German pathologist T. Frerichs showed that black particles consisted of degraded hemoglobin. The Italian scientists Angelo Celli and Ettore Manchiafava first coined the word "*Plasmodium*" for the parasite they found. From 1884 to 1885, they examined hundreds of fresh and stained blood slides that enabled them to assemble a series of motion pictures which highlighted the parasite's feeding habits and the accumulation of black pigment. A Cuban doctor named Carlos Finlay a year later proved that yellow fever was transmitted by mosquitoes and transmitted the disease between humans. Camillo Golgi also contributed to the field by confirming that all the parasites in the blood divided simultaneously and at regular intervals. He also showed, after studying the series of blood slides, that a new generation of quartan parasites which is now recognized as *P malariae* appeared every 72 hours.

In 1898, Britain's Sir Ronald Ross, working in the Presidency General Hospital in Calcutta India, finally established that malaria was transmitted by mosquitoes after he found that certain mosquito species transmit malaria to birds. He did this after isolating the parasites from the salivary glands of the mosquito that had then fed on the infected birds. He was awarded the Nobel Prize for Medicine in 1902. After he left India, Sir Ross joined the newly established Liverpool School of Tropical Medicine and supervised the efforts to control malaria in Egypt, Greece, Mauritius and Panama. In 1900, the works of Finlay and Ross were confirmed by a medical board headed by Walter Reed. Dr. Patrick Manson worked on the theory that malaria might be transmitted by mosquitoes and historical evidence showed that he worked closely with Ross. One person who played a part in the malaria effort was an Italian named Giovanni Battista Grassi. He is acknowledged also for revealing that mosquitoes transmit human malaria. There is even the argument that he was unjustly overlooked for the 1902 Nobel Prize.

Malaria was first treated effectively with the bark of the cinchona tree which contains quinine. The tree is mostly found on the slopes of the Andes, primarily in Peru where the inhabitants used a tincture made from the bark of the tree to control malaria. The active ingredient, quinine, was extracted and isolated by two French chemists, Pierre Joseph Pelletier and Joseph Binaime Caventou. The story of the tree has it that a Spanish countess of Chinchon traveled to Peru. While there she contracted a fever which was cured with the bark. When she returned to Spain, she brought the bark which she introduced to Europe in 1638. In 1742, a botanist, Carl Linnaeus named the tree "Chinchona" in her honor. In the early 20th century before antibiotics became available, Julius Wagner-Jauregg discovered that patients with syphilis could be treated by intentionally infecting them with malaria. The resulting fever killed the spirochetes and then the quinine was administered to control the malaria.

The Italian Parliament passed a series of laws between 1900 and 1907 establishing national campaign efforts to either eradicate or at least control malaria. This was significant in that it was the first campaign of its kind in the world. A range of efforts were initiated focusing on mosquito control, microscopic diagnosis of malaria and quinine treatment resulting in the elimination of malaria in all of Western Europe by the mid- 1930s. In 1936, the League of Nations Pan-African Health conference was held which concluded that Africa received far less malaria control than did other parts of the world and that the future success of malaria control depended on the economic improvement of Africans. This was important because at that time the colonial powers only believed in grabbing Africa's vast resources.

Dichlor-diphenyl-trichloroethane (DDT) was discovered in 1939 which revolutionized malaria control through spraying. This led to the development of the indoor residual spraying technique (IRS) which required only two or three applications on indoor surfaces in a year. The effect was the dramatic reduction in malaria transmission that was experienced in the Balkans, Mexico, Latin America, Sri Lanka, Taiwan, the Middle East and Greece. In the 1940s, as part of its effort, the United States Army 2nd World War Drug Development program made chloroquine available as the first synthetic antimalarial drug with an acceptable tolerability and safety profile that could be mass produced. These provided the necessary weapons for new malaria control efforts. Most of the progress attained in the fight against malaria was however undone by World War II. This was attributed to infrastructure losses and massive population displacement. In the aftermath of the Second World War was the formation of the United Nations (UN) on 24 October 1945. This was followed in 1948 with the formation of its specialized organization for health issues, the World Health Organization (WHO). Malaria was one of the early topics of discussion for the WHO Interim Committee. The first session of the WHO malaria expert committee was held in April 1947. By early 1950, the first report of Anopheles resistant to DDT was reported followed by *Plasmodium falciparum* resistance to chloroquine which spread to all areas with *falciparum* malaria by the 1980s.

With these setbacks, the world was faced with a dilemma. If the effective control methods were to be rendered useless, what would be the next strategy? This created some sense of urgency since the window of opportunity was very narrow. One issue at that time was identifying the role of DDT. This raised a fierce argument between the advocates for malaria control using IRS with DDT and the proponents of the general health improvement technique. In 1950, the WHO Conference in Africa was held in Kampala and delegates identified that malaria had a negative effect on the development of Africa and there was a need to attack the malaria burden to ensure large scale development in Africa. In 1955, the WHO launched the Global Malaria Eradication Program (GMEP) with the aim of launching an all-out war on malaria through the use of a uniformly single approach to target areas. They anticipated that rigorous use of IRS with DDT or even other insecticides in combination with malaria case detection and treatment would bring malaria down to such a level that the remaining few cases could be dealt with through surveillance.

The ultimate goal was the global eradication of malaria. The WHO regional committees approved this approach with the exception of the Africa Regional Committee which argued that preparation needed for effective IRS implementation was not yet available and there was no documented evidence to show that surveillance was adequate in a region with a high incidence of transmission. At the 2nd Africa Malaria Conference in Lagos in November 1955, delegates considered that the physical, economic and developmental challenges in Africa in combination with the high endemicity as well as prolonged transmission made it prudent to temporarily exclude Africa from the general proposals for the eradication of malaria as touted by the World Health Assembly. In 1956, a Malaria Eradication Special Account was established to help sustain the eradication effort. Over 44 countries contributed about US$20.33 million within seven years with the US contributing over 85% of the total. In 1969, when it was at the height of its effort, GMEP activities covered about 1.4 billion people which were about 40% of the 3.6 billion world population at the time. In 1969, it was also recognized that there was the need to change the global malaria eradication effort from a time-limited campaign to a long-term goal. The strategy started focusing on control. However, in reality, the approach depended on the treatment of the febrile phase of the disease.

During the 1970s and 1980s, malaria associated mortality was alarmingly high due to the spread of chloroquine resistance. In the mid 1970's, the WHO, joined later by the United Nations Development Program (UNDP), World Bank, and UNICEF launched the Special Program for Research and Training (TDR) which developed a series of activities in malaria medicine, epidemiology and immunology including a search for a malaria vaccine. With funding for malaria dwindling and the attention focused on other issues, malaria made a dramatic return in the so-called epidemic 'rebound' in areas that GMEP had managed to almost eradicate malaria. At the 1978 International Conference on Primary Healthcare, the Alma Ata Declaration was adopted resulting in the World Health Assembly adopting a new malaria control strategy for malaria mortality reduction using an epidemiological approach with the ultimate goal being eradication, if possible. The variants used for this strategy were: 1. Reduction and prevention of mortality due to malaria; 2. Reduction and prevention of mortality and morbidity particularly in high-risk groups; 3. Reduction of the prevalence and endemicity of malaria; and 4. Countrywide malaria control aimed at eradication.

By the early 1990s, it was obvious that the control of malaria was becoming a failure which was considered to be a disaster. A meeting was organized in 1992 in Amsterdam, Netherlands with the aim of refocusing global attention on malaria. It resulted in the launching of a global declaration on the control of malaria with Africa being very prominent. The meeting expressed the need for an urgent commitment to malaria control by all stake holders. In 1995, the UN Secretary-General launched a special initiative for Africa which made malaria control one of its specific goals. Even though the malaria control effort was then faltering amid severe criticism, it must be stated that international advocacy had some wonderful success. In 1998, global spending on malaria was around US$100 million. This increased, however, to $5.3 billion by the end of 2009 covering 191 malaria grants in 82 countries. The fund was used to support prioritized interventions across most African countries. These interventions included insecticide-treated nets, reduction of maternal and neonatal effect of malaria infection during pregnancy, selective use of indoor residual house spraying as well as the replacement of failing drugs with artemisinin-based combination therapy (ACT) and improvement of point of care using rapid tests. The 1990s saw the global efforts on malaria control turned towards Africa resulting in the development of a series of initiatives such as the Global Malaria Control Strategy formulated after a series of consultations and interregional conferences during 1991 and 1992. This was ratified in October 1992. A WHO program for accelerated implementation of malaria control in Africa was established in 1997.

Table 1. Global Malaria Action Plan Objective (approved by RBM Partnership Board 2011)

Objective 1: Reduce global malaria deaths to near zero by end 2015.
Objective 2: Reduce global cases by 75% by the end of 2015 (from 2000 levels)
Objective 3:Eliminate malaria by the end of 2015 in at least 8 to 10 countries including the entire World Health Organization European Region

In 1998, the Roll Back Malaria (RBM) initiative was launched with its objectives outlined in Table 1. It identified the four main strategies need to achieve the RBM 'dream' as: 1. Prompt access to effective treatment; 2. Malaria prevention through vector control especially using ITNs; 3. Prevention and management of malaria in pregnancy; and 4. Prevention of and effective response to malaria in epidemic and complex emergencies. The main focus of RBM was Africa.

In April 2000, Africa leaders met for the Africa Summit on Roll Back Malaria where the famous Abuja Declaration on Roll Back Malaria in Africa was signed. Among the remarkable statements of the declaration were:

- Malaria is a barrier to development and poverty alleviation in Africa.
- Malaria has slowed economic growth in Africa countries to the extent that some countries were experiencing a negative growth rate.

To address the malaria menace, the leaders requested that:

- The debt of poor and heavily indebted nations in Africa should be canceled in order to release resources for poverty alleviation and RBM.
- Allocation of substantial new resources of at least US$1 billion per year to RBM in Africa.

This resulted in international donors such as the World Bank pledging an additional US$300-500 million towards malaria control in Africa. CIDA donated an additional US$6.5 million over a period of 5 years towards RBM in Africa. A technical consultation meeting was held in Rabat, Morocco in 2002 which resulted in the formulation of the 1st WHO guidelines on malaria elimination. Most significantly, the malaria genome was released in 2002. This was an important landmark in malaria medicine since it provided scientists with the tool to scientifically study malaria properly. In 2003, four countries in Africa adopted ACTs as their first-line treatment of malaria. However, by 2010, it had become the first-line treatment in all African countries where malaria was endemic. In 2005, the Global Fund to Fight AIDS, Tuberculosis and Malaria was established with the aim of providing large scale funding for health related Millennium Development Goals (MDG). With the issues of both changes in malaria and invasive bacterial diseases taking place side by side, there was a need to change the strategy.

The achievement on the island of Bioko, Equatorial Guinea is worth mentioning. In 2003, an integrated malaria control program was initiated. After four years, there was major reduction in the entomological variants of transmission which led to a massive reduction in the rate of parasitemia and anemia; with a two-third reduction in malaria associated mortality among children under the age of five being the most significant. Taking into consideration such an accomplishment, it was concluded that Bioko was able to achieve its MDG for childhood mortality in single year through a single system. We can reason from this that Bioko with its small population was able to achieve this feat. Why can't we implement similar programs in larger populations? In October 2007, Seattle, Washington, USA hosted a meeting which completely transformed the framework of the global malaria control strategy with the aim being "eradication of malaria". Table 2 chronicles some of the events that assisted in improving malaria medicine.

Table 2. Recent milestone in malaria research

Year	Finding	Reference
2002	Release of malaria genome	Gardner MJ et al. 2002
2003	Malaria transcriptome described	Bozdech Z et al., 2003
2004	RTS,S efficacious in children	Alonso PL, et al. 2004
2005	A study of the prevalence in Africa children started	
2007	Chaperone network described	Pavithra SR et al., 2007
2008	RTS,S phase II clinical trial commence	
2009	A study revealed the presence of core interactome in *P falciparum*	Wuchty S, et al., 2009
2010	Signaling transduction pathway in malaria Spiroindolines described as potential antimalaria agents	Oyelade J, et al. 2010 Rottamann M, et al. 2010
2011	Identification of basigin receptor	Grosnier C, et al. 2011
2011	1st result of RTS,S	RTS,S partnership
2013	GSK announces that it will apply for approval for 1st malaria vaccine registration	www.rsc.org

Evolution of Malaria Parasite

Where did the malaria parasites evolve from? An attempt is made to trace the origin of the malaria parasite with the questions of when, where and how did they enter the human population. Before addressing these questions, the main polymorphism found in human genetics which plays a role in the malaria hypothesis will be discussed.

Thalassemias

These are a class of anemia associated with abnormalities in the gene coding for hemoglobin. It involves the effective loss of either the alpha (alpha-thalassemia) or beta (beta-thalassemia) chain of the molecule. Many specific mutations in the genes for the alpha and beta hemoglobin chains have been described among the known thalassemias. Numerous studies have shown and proven that there is an association between thalassemia and a long standing exposure of a population to the presence of malaria. This was initially determined by Halden. This was further confirmed in studies which showed that in Africa, the Arabian Peninsula, Middle East, Central Asia, Islands of the Western Pacific, New Guinea and the islands of Melanesia there are high frequencies of thalassemias whereas in Europe, high frequencies are found on the shore of the Mediterranean Sea. The reduction in the risk of malarial diseases has been shown to be associated with heretozygotes and homozygotes for certain $alpha^{+}$ thalassemias.

Glucose-6-Phosphate Deficiency

This is due to a mutation in the sex-linked gene for glucose-6-phosphate dehydrogenases (G6PD) giving rise to G6PD deficiencies. It was first identified in a condition referred to as favism as a result of a hemolytic crisis in those affected after the consumption of oxidant food like fava beans. G6PD is now recognized as a hazard in high risk malaria regions because taking antimalaria drugs such as primaquine is associated with oxidant stress. Studies have shown that the combination of hemizygous and heterozygous in G6PD deficiency is associated with a high level of protection against severe *P falciparum*. This means that a high rate of G6PD deficiency in many parts of the world can be attributed to selection by malaria. Tishkoff et al. showed that alleles for G6PD deficiencies were diagnosed in Africans between 4,000 and 12,000 years ago. This was the period which some estimated that *P falciparum* might have emerged as a major human pathogen. It is believed that selection for G6PD deficiency might have preceded this event and an overlap occurred at a time when *P vivax* could had been a major selective force in Africa.

Sickle Cell Trait

Thalassemias and G6PD deficiency reduces the risk of death from *P falciparum* by about 50%. However, certain human mutations have been identified that provide at least 90% protection from malaria-linked mortality. Among these is the gene for sickle cell hemoglobin (Hemoglobin C). The sickle cell trait is the result of a single point mutation in the gene for the beta chain of the hemoglobin where glutamate found in position 6 is replaced with valine. This leads to a hemoglobin molecule, Hemoglobin C. In its homozygote form, gives rise to sickle cell anemia. It has been confirmed that such a mutation offers protection against the risk of death from *P falciparum* malaria. Children in West Africa who are heterozygous for the sickle cell gene have been found to have a 1/10 risk of death from *P falciparum* malaria compared to children who are homozygous for the normal gene. In many parts of Africa, the frequency of the sickle cell gene exceeds 30%.

Hemoglobin C

The hemoglobin C gene is allelic to the sickle cell hemoglobin but it codes for a lysine instead of a glutamate (Hemoglobin H) or a valine (Hemoglobin S) at position 6 in the beta chain of the hemoglobin molecule. In the homozygous carriers, it confers loss of fitness which is less than those associated with the sickle cell trait. Hemoglobin C is found only among certain segments of the West African population where its frequency reaches up to 10 to 20%. There have been some arguments about this mutation and whether it is still being selected in West Africa under the effect of *P falciparum* malaria. Its nature of protection differs from those associated with hemoglobin S. While in hemoglobin S, the heterozygous form confers a high level of protection against *P falciparum* malaria deaths, in hemoglobin C a similar level of protection, greater than 90% against infection and subsequent death by *P falciparum* are achieved only in the homozygote form.

The next step is to analyze this from an evolutionary perspective. The rate of selection of an allele whose advantage is expressed mainly in homozygous forms like in hemoglobin C is slow when compared to that of an allele which carries a similar advantage but in heterozygous form like hemoglobin S. Under any influence of the same selective force, hemoglobin S would be expected to achieve higher frequencies than hemoglobin C. Because the balance of cost of hemoglobin C is low while that of hemoglobin S is high, hemoglobin C is expected to replace hemoglobin S in the population which has been exposed to *P falciparum*. In West Africa, this has not yet happened which suggests that *falciparum* malaria might have arrived in the West African population recently. But how recent is that? The relative finesses of the different hemoglobin alleles have been described while the relative calculations have been made. It is suspected that the hemoglobin C allele should approach population equilibrium within several thousand years and certainly less than tens of thousands of years due to selection from *P falciparum.* From this argument, it can be assumed that because hemoglobin C has not yet reached its expected equilibrium, *P falciparum* has been a selective force in West Africa less than this time with a suggested time frame of a few tens of thousands years ago.

Hemoglobin E

The replacement of glutamate in position 26 of the beta chain in hemoglobin A, leads to hemoglobin E, found to occur at high frequencies in the people of Southeast Asia. It has no clinical effects but in combination with certain thalassemia mutations it does have some effect. It does not impose any cost on a carrier. There has not been any reports which highlight any protection against *P falciparum* infection. However, studies have shown that it might protect against *P vivax* infection. Other studies have reported that hemoglobin train patients are capable of clearing *P falciparum* more rapidly than certain drug treatments with artemisinin derivatives. It has also been established that the regions where hemoglobin E is prevalent also have the most malaria cases. Therefore, the burden of malaria in these regions has been one of the heaviest in the world. This means from the malaria hypothesis point of view, the gene for hemoglobin E is an absolute good candidate for selection under the pressure of malaria, possibly under *P vivax*. Based on this principle, it can be argued that this selection took place prior to the arrival of *P falciparum* in this population.

Ovalocytosis

This is a type of polymorphism that affects the main structural protein of RBCs known as band 3. Mutations as a result of a deletion in the gene for this protein have been identified as a genetic determinant of ovalocytosis which occurs due to an abnormal shape of affected RBCs in the heterozygote. It appears there is no homozygote for band 3 deletion. This type of mutation is found in Melanesia beyond the Indonesian and Malay inhabited archipelago on the Western Pacific rim. This also includes the Islands of New Guinea, the Solomon Island and the Island of Vanuatu. In this region, malaria transmission is among the highest. This explains why there is high frequency of ovalocytosis in this populace. Ovalocytosis is very frequent; up to 20% in the highly malarious lowlands of New Guinea but found to be completely absent in the malaria-free highlands. Carriers of this genetic trait are at reduced risk of being infected by *P falciparum* and *P vivax* malaria.

RBC Duffy Negativity

The Duffy antigen is encoded by the FY gene and is also known as the Duffy antigen receptor for chemokine (DARC). It plays a role in chemokine regulation and has been a receptor for human susceptibility to *P vivax* and *P knowlesi* in some non-human primates. Several results have shown that people who lack the Duffy antigen are naturally protected from *P vivax* malaria. Most West Africans and 68% of African Americans do not express the Duffy antigen subtypes FY*A and FY*B in their red blood cells. The nucleic acid variants in GATA-1 found in the gene promoter is responsible for the non expression of the Duffy antigen on the RBCs, subsequently leading to resistance to invasion by *P vivax*. The Duffy antigen subtypes also can also be found in different form as a mutant or null as FY*A ^{null} or FY*B ^{null}. In addition to being a chemokine receptor, the Duffy antigen is also an important receptor for *P vivax* merozoites which enables the parasite to enter the host RBCs.

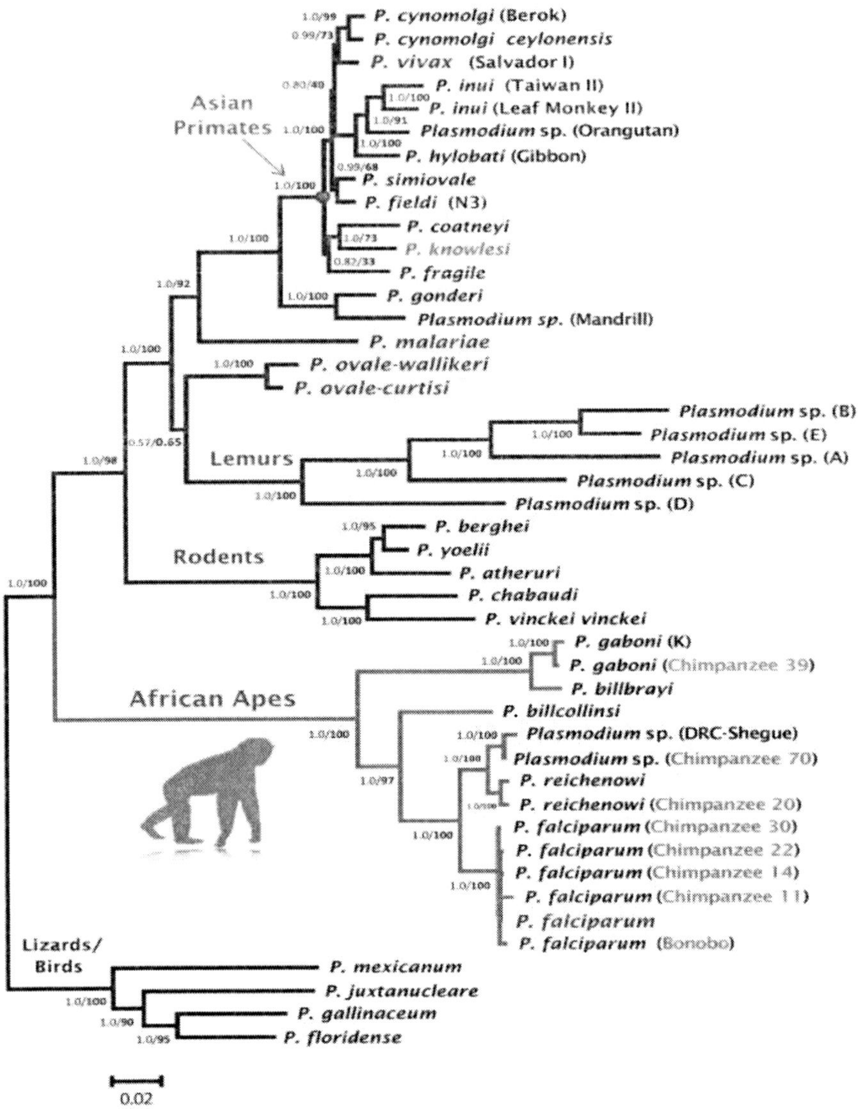

Figure 1. Evolutionary trend among P falciparum-associated parasites from apes, humans and monkeys. (Adopted from Pacheco et al.)

Where, When and How Did Malaria Evolved?

Plasmodium is found in a broad range of vertebrate hosts which includes mammals, birds and reptiles. Molecular phylogenetic analysis has proven that host switches are common in these parasites as shown in regards to *P falciparum* which clustered with two avian parasites instead of those infecting mammals. This suggests that *P falciparum* was due to the transfer from birds to humans. It is believed that this might have taken place about 10,000 years ago when human habitat settled. The four species of *Plasmodium* do not form a monophyletic group but instead are part of two distinct clades of primate malarias. One of the clades is made up of *P vivax, P ovale* and *P malariae* with other several *Plasmodium* species found in non-human primates while a second clade which includes *P falciparum* and other lineages are found in African apes. Molecular phylogenetic studies have further shown that the *Plasmodium* species might have originated 4 to 7 million years ago. The belief is that non-human primates might have been introduced into Southeast Asia by a non-Homindae primate where they were then passed on through an explosive species radiation process. These might have had a series of host switches which involved switching that allowed the colonization of humans by the lineage that originated from *P vivax*. However, there is no evidence to prove that the falciparum-like parasite was found in Asian non-human primates. Based on this finding, the accepted hypothesis is that *P vivax* originated from Asia while *P falciparum* came from Africa. There has been some argument recently about this model. For example, lineages of African *P vivax* have been described in chimpanzees and humans. But molecular data has shown that they were introduced into Africa posteriori. If we accept the Asian and African model of originality, the next question is how did the evolution take place? Studies have shown that *P falciparum* is closer to *P reichenowi* which is found in chimpanzees. Escalante and Ayala have suggested that these two parasites diverged during the divergence phase between humans and chimpanzees. Their results showed that *P falciparum* did not originate directly from an avian malaria parasite. However, *P falciparum* and *P reichenowi* are considered as a sister lineage from birds and lizards.

Subsequent studies presented contrasting views. There were those who argued that *P falciparum/ P reichenowi* clade was added simply because they were included in the mammalian group and were closer to rodent or primate *Plasmodium*. There were others who were of the view that they clustered closely with parasites from birds. This confusion arose because there were biases while representing certain taxa. In 2008, Martinesen et al. concluded that *P falciparum* can be placed at the basal of all other mammalian malaria parasite. By adding more taxa from primates, the origin of *P falciparum* was firmly established. For example, Ollomo et al. in 2009 outlined the complete mitochondrial genome of a new species which had earlier not been described. These species of *Plasmodium* were found to be circulating in great apes and belonged to the *P falciparum/ P reichenowi* lineage. This species was called *P gaboni* because they were discovered in wild-borne chimpanzees which were kept as pets in a village in Gabon. Taking into consideration that there was a hypothesis of *P falciparum* and *P reichenowi* having diverged about 6 million years ago, Ollomo et al. concluded that the ancestor of this African great apes/ human parasite clade might have been present in hominid ancestors. A study by Liu et al. also showed the existence of six *Plasmodium* species which belonged to the *Laverania* subgenus of which three were found in chimpanzees and three in gorillas. The former they called C1-C3 while the later were called G1-G3. The study gave a more definite picture of *Laverania* associated diversity. This finding supports the hypothesis that the likely origin of *P falciparum* is the gorilla. In contrast, Prugnolle et al. reported that after amplifying *P falciparum* sequence from the blood of a pet monkey, they proposed that their "finding challenges the gorilla origin of the human strain of *P falciparum*". However, the conclusion cannot be justified from the data presented. Further studies need to be undertaken to confirm or dispute these studies. The remaining species, *P vivax, P malariae* and *P ovale* are within a single clade which includes all mammalian malaria parasites other than *P falciparum* and *P reichenowi*. The three seem to have diverged about 100 million years ago. *P ovale* is known to be an infection and no genetically close relative has been described. This makes it the sole known survivor representing its line. *P malariae*, apart from infecting humans, is also found to be a natural parasite of chimpanzees in West Africa. A morphologically similar parasite *P brazilianum* has been found to infect New World monkeys in Central and South America. However, molecular analysis failed to differentiate between *P malariae* and *P brazilianum*. It is possible that these are the same or almost the same parasites infecting humans and New World monkeys. From this perspective, one can argue that *P brazilianum* is a zoonotic form of *P malariae* which was recently introduced from humans to New World monkey populations. Some have, however, argued that there was instead a lateral transfer from New World monkeys to humans. *P brazilianum* is the only known lineage with *P malariae*. *P vivax,* on the other hand, belong to a closely related and large body of malaria parasites which have been described to infect mainly monkeys of Southern and Southeastern Asia as well as the Western Pacific zone. Molecular analysis has placed *P cynomolgi* as closely related to *P vivax*. The prevalent view is that *P vivax* might have originated from the Southern Asian regions because most of the close relatives have been found infecting monkeys in that region. It is possible that *P vivax* and *P cynomolgi* might have diverged about two to three million years ago. The scientific community has a challenging question to tackle: Are there other Plasmodia species out there? Figure 1 outlines the evolutionary journey of *Plasmodium*.

Chapter II

The Malaria Parasite and Its Life Cycle

Human malaria is caused by four species of *Plasmodium*: *P. falciparum*, *P. vivax*, and *P. ovales* and *P malariae*. However, the latest evidence implicates a fifth species, *P. knowlesi* (which was initially thought to infect only non-human primates) in human malaria infection. The malaria parasite has a complicated life cycle which alternates between a sporogenic stage which occurs in the female Anopheles mosquito and two stages that are found in the human host: inside the liver, referred to as the exo-erythrocytic stage and within the blood which is referred to as the erythrocytic stage. The malaria cycle (Figure 2) begins when the female Anopheles mosquito bites a victim and the sporozoites found in the infected mosquito's salivary gland are introduced through the bridged skin during the process of feeding by the mosquito. From the skin, they make their way to the liver. Studies have shown that this takes only a matter of minutes. In the liver, the sporozoites are transformed to schizonts. Within 48 hours, thousands of merozoites develop within each schizont.

The rupturing of the hepatoctytes results in the invasion of the red blood cells (RBCs) by the merozoites where they undergo asexual multiplication. Within the RBCs, the merozoites initially grow into a ring-shaped form then into a larger form of trophozoite. This is transformed into the schizont stage during which the parasite divides several times resulting in the production of new merozoites. This then bursts from this cell to invade new RBCs in a well defined periodic pattern which lasts between two to three days. This stage normally takes place two to three weeks after the host has been bitten by the infected mosquito. The asexual phase continues until it is controlled either by the use of drugs or immune response or death of the patient in the case of *P falciparum*. After the invasion of the RBCs, some of the merozoites differentiate into gametocytes (sexual forms). When these are taken in by the female Anopheles mosquito, they mature into male and female gametes in the blood meal. After fertilization, a zygote is formed which matures within 24 hours to form an ookinete in the mosquito mid-gut. It burrows its way to and encysts on the basal lamina. Further development over a two week period results in the formation of oocysts full of sporozoites. When the oocysts rupture, the sporozoites are released and they migrate to the salivary glands through the hemocoel. In the salivary glands, the sporozoites can remain latent for some weeks and still maintain their viability. The injection of these sporozoites sparks another episode of new infection. It has been suggested that the meiotic division and sexual process allows genetic recombination to take place. The proteome analysis of the various stages of the malaria parasite has revealed the presence of a series of proteins; 315 malaria proteins are found solely in gametocytes, 226 in trophozoites and schizonts and 97 in gametes. A total of 575 proteins were described in the sexual stage (gametocytes and gametes) 488 proteins in both sexual and asexual stages.

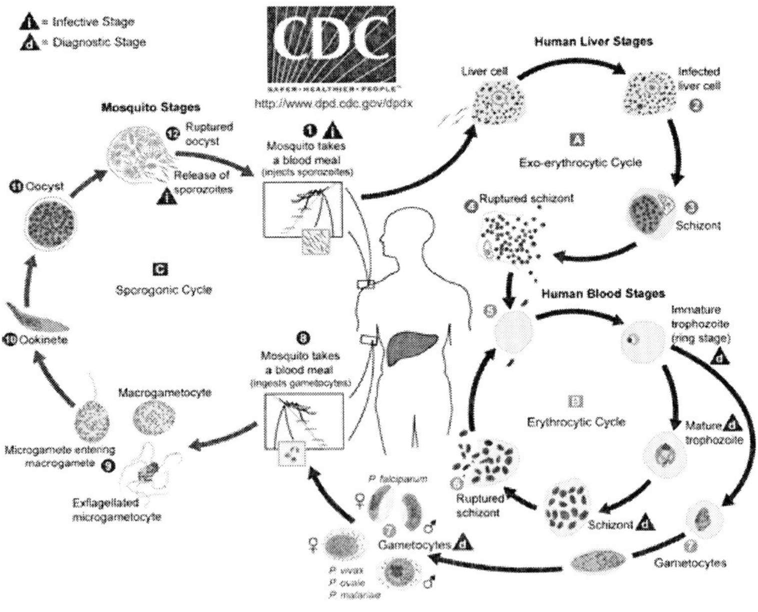

Figure 2. The malaria parasite life cycle. (Credit: CDC)

Brief Insight into Plasmodium Genome

The *P falciparum* genome is made up of 22.8 megabase (Mb) distributed among 14 chromosomes which range in size from 0.643 to 3.29Mb. It has been found that the *P falciparum* genome is twice the size of the *Schizosaccharomyces pombe* genome. The genome of *P falciparum* and several of the *Plasmodium* species are unusual because they show some biasness toward two nucleotides: adenine (A) and Thymine (T). In the region coding for proteins, the A+T bias is greater than 76% while in the intergenic region and introns, the A+T content can reach 100%. This extreme biasness has been linked to difficulty in cloning and maintaining large segments of *P falciparum* DNA in *E coli.* In all, the A+T composition is 80.6% which rises to approximately 90% in introns and intergenic regions. About 5,300 protein-encoding genes have been identified. It has been suggested that the gene density in *P falciparum* is about 1 gene per 4,338 base pairs (bp). When one excludes the intron, the mean length of the *P falciparum* gene is 2.3kb making it larger than in other organisms with the average gene length between 1.3 to 1.6 kb. In addition, the *P falciparum* genes have a remarkably greater proportion of genes which are about 15.5% longer when compared to *S pombe* and *S cerevisiae* which are about 3.0% and 3.6% respectively. Many of the large genes encode for some uncharacterized proteins that may be cystolic proteins because they do not possess any recognizable signal peptides. In addition, no transposable elements or retrotransposons have been identified. 52% of the predicted gene products (2,731) have been detected in several stages of the life cycle of the parasite. These include many predicted genes which are not similar to other proteins in other organisms. It has also been found that 49% of the genes overlap with expressed sequence tags (ESTs) which are derived from several stages in the lifecycle. The nuclear genome contains a full set of transfer RNA (tRNA) ligase genes of which 43 have been found to bind all codons except TGT and TGC, coding for Cys. It has been suggested that these tRNAs are located within an unsequenced region. A putative selenoprotein was found which may provide selenium for selenoproteins synthesis. It has been observed that there is an increase in growth in selenium supplemented *Plasmodium* culture. The tRNA genes of almost all eukaryotes exhibit some range of redundancy except the intracellular parasite *Encephalitozoon cunicul*i which has been found to contain 44tRNAs. Further studies have revealed that the abundance of specific anticodons is correlated with the codon use of the organism. However, in *P falciparum*, there is minimal redundancy of tRNAs. The reason for this is that the mitochondrial genome of *Plasmodium* is small. It is about 6kb which does not encode tRNAs, so the mitochondrion has to import tRNAs. The malaria genome does not contain the long tandem repeated arrays which are seen in other eukaryotes. Instead, the parasite contains several single 18S-5.8S-28S rRNA units found distributed on different chromosomes. The rRNA gene encoding sequence in one unit is different from the sequence of the corresponding rRNA in other units. It has also been found that expression of each rRNA unit is regulated during development resulting in the expression of different rRNAs during different stages of the *Plasmodium* life cycle. It has been suggested that changing the properties of its ribosome enables the parasite to change its rate of translation, either specific messenger RNAs (mRNAs) which enable it to change the rate of cell growth or the pattern of cell development. Earlier, 2 types of rRNA genes were described in *P falciparum* as S-type which are mostly present in the mosquito vector and A-type which are present in the human host. In the genome sequence, seven loci which encode rRNAs have been identified. Two copies of the S-type rRNA gene have been located on chromosome 11 and 13 while in the A-type, on chromosome 5 and 7.

Metabolism: An Overview

The malaria parasite has a rapid growth and multiplication rate during most of the stages of its life cycle. This means that the parasite requires nutrients and metabolizes these into various biological molecules to enable it to survive and reproduce. A brief description of these processes in *Plasmodia* is presented below.

Biochemical studies of the malaria parasite have been limited to the intra-erythrocytic stage of its life cycle because of the difficulty in finding a suitable amount of material from other stages of its life cycle. In the erythrocytic stage, *P falciparum* relies on anaerobic glycolysis for the production of energy by the regeneration of NAD^+ through the conversion of pyruvate to lactate. Genes which encode the enzyme needed for functional glycolytic pathway have been identified. They include a phosphofructokinase (PFK) whose sequence is similar to the pyrophosphate- dependent group of enzymes but there is the suggestion that it is probably ATP-dependent because of the characterization of the homologous enzyme in *P berghei*. A pyrophosphate-dependent PFK which possesses an N- and carboxyl-terminal extension is also present which could represent the target sequences. Studies could not identify any gene encoding for fructose bisphosphatase which suggest that gluconeogenesis is absent. Enzymes for the synthesis of trehalose, glycogen and carbohydrate are also absent. Candidate genes required for the convention of pentose phosphate pathways have been identified. These include bifunctional glucose-6 phosphate dehydrogenase/6-phosphoglucose-6 dehydrogenases which are needed for NADPH as well as ribose-5-phosphate required for other biosynthetic pathways. Erythrose-4 – phosphate needed for chorismata pathway has also been described and it is believed to generate from the glycolytic intermediate fructose-6-phosphate and glyceraldehydes 3-phosphate through a putative transkelolase. However, transaldolase seems to be absent. The Tricarboxylic acid cycle (TCA) is the central point of carbon metabolism serving to connect the processes of glycolysis, gluconeogenesis, respiration, synthesis of amino acid and other biosynthetic pathways.

Several genes have been identified which are needed to complete a TCA cycle. An important de novo heme biosynthesis pathway was identified which implies that Succinly-Coenzyme (Succinly-CoA) is generated in the mitochondrion. A study reported on the intracellular levels of several TCA metabolites which rotate in the parasite growth cycle in stages which support the expression of profiles of cognate enzymes. It has therefore been suggested that TCA metabolites are actively synthesized by the parasite. A pyruvate dehydrogenase was found but it still remains unclear whether the TCA cycle is used for the oxidation of glycolysis products or to supply intermediate products for other biosynthetic pathways. Pyruvate dehydrogenase (PDH) complex is localized not in the mitochondrion but in the apicoplast, a non-photosynthetic plastid-like organelle. The PDH has been suggested to produce acetyl-Coenzyme A (acetyl-CoA) which is only used for fatty acid elongation. A similar protein aconitases has been reported to be the cytosolic iron-response elements binding protein which does not possess aconitase activity. Genes are also present that encode malate-quinone oxidoreductase which appears to be linked to the mitochondria. It is believed that this replaces malate dehydrogenase in the TCA cycle. All of these findings suggest the existence of an active mitochondrial pathway. There is a gene present that encodes phosphoenolpyruvate (PEPC). Just as in bacteria, *P falciparum* is able to cope with drain exhaustion. This is supported by findings that the incorporation of carbon dioxide activity takes place in the sexual stage of the parasite in culture. It was proposed that an unusual TCA cycle may be operating in the essential stage of *P falciparum* fuelled by the catabolism of glutamine via the built in oxidative and reductive arms of the TCA cycle. However, this proposal was retracted. It has also been suggested that the operation of a complete mitochondrial TCA cycle is not required for the development of the asexual stage in a murine related parasite *P berghei.* The extent to which a conventional or unconventional TCA cycle operates in *P falciparum* RBC stages is still unclear. Despite the absence of recognized mitochondrial PDH in P falciparum, increasing evidence points to the fact that the conventional TCA cycle can operate in the insect stage of these parasites or other apicomplexan parasites. The data presented shows that the TCA cycle is essential for the growth of intracellular stage of *Toxoplasma gondii.* A study showed that both the asexual and sexual blood stages of the *P falciparum* utilize a conventional TCA cycle to catabolize glucose and glutamine thereby suggesting that there should be a review of the current model of *P falciparum* carbon metabolism. In addition, it was shown that gametocyte differentiation is associated with a programmed remodeling of the central carbon metabolism that maybe required for parasite survival either before or after uptake by a mosquito vector. Since the TCA cycle plays a central role in the life cycle of the malaria parasite, more studies need to be conducted to understand the molecular mechanism of activities associated with it which might lead to the development of transmission-blocking drugs.

Metabolomics in Malaria Research

Metabolomics is the process of profiling a set of metabolites or lower molecular weight biochemical metabolites due to the physiological, developmental or pathological processes in cells, tissues, organs or organisms. Metabolomics is emerging as an exciting field in infectious diseases research which is leading to the development of new, more accurate databases, complex bioinformatics software and spectral libraries. A series of techniques combine to make this field exciting including: ligand and gas chromatography, genome sequencing, mass spectrometry, nuclear magnetic resonance spectrometry and MS/MS spectral libraries. Metabolomics has been used for the identification of biomarkers, diagnosis, classification of diseases, understanding the mechanism of drug action and toxicity, analyzing the biochemical function of metabolites flux and regulation mechanisms. The anti-drug resistance in malaria is a major public health problem which requires studies to identify the key drug targets. Metabolomics can provide that platform. In addition, Metabolomics present an opportunity to study host-parasite interactions in malaria infection which hopefully, will open the avenue for prospective malaria vaccine development. Others have utilized the concept of Metabolomics in malaria research. Olszewski et al. in a study which first utilized the concept of Metabolomics for *P falciparum* using the LC-MS analytical platform, measured the relative levels of about 80 metabolites in cell extracts and culture mediums and reported many alterations to the host cell. They also found a novel metabolic phenotype in that the *Plasmodium* parasite quickly and specifically degraded extracellular arginine into non-proteogenic amino acids ornithine. This is a reaction that they determined to be catalyzed by the *P falciparum* arginase enzyme. It is postulated that this may be a correlation between clinical hypoarginane and malaria infection. Further study would aid in understanding the mechanism of the action of poorly characterized antimalaria drugs and the metabolic correlation of drug-resistant mutation. Another interesting study by Sana et al. used Metabolomics to profile in vitro P falciparum-infected (IRBC) and uninfected (NRBC) erythrocytes reported of over-representation of many metabolites onto several IRBC pathways especially glycolysis. Furthermore, they found that components of branched TCA cycle; partial urea cycle, nucleotides, amino acids, chorismates, sphingolipids and fatty acids metabolisms were altered in IRBCs. They also identified and confirmed an elevated level of cyclic ADP ribose and phosphoribosyl AMP in IRBC. Several compounds have been identified which were initially not associated with P falciparum; such as PRib-AMP and cADPR which are both adenine-containing nucleotides and were studied in mammalian systems. Metabolomics can be used to identify key metabolic pathways which can be used as novel drug and vaccine targets.

Chapter III

Recent Advances in the Epidemiology of Human Malaria

Molecular Epidemiology

Introduction

In the past, apart from a microscope, epidemiologists had few tools to study malaria and infectious diseases in general. However, during the past few years, two new techniques have been introduced that are being used in the epidemiological study of infectious diseases with huge success. Data can now be used to accurately map the distribution of malaria, while the prevalence rate can accurately be matched to its variables such as climate, population density, etc using a geographical information system (GIS). In the laboratory, the use of the now more effective polymerase chain reaction (PCR) has made the study of the malaria parasite, its host and vectors possible. This has improved the epidemiological data that is now available.

Polymerase Chain Reaction

The Polymerase Chain Reaction (PCR) is a biochemical method that involves synthesizing millions of copies of a specific sequence of DNA (target sequence). It was initially described by Kary Mullis in 1983 and has since become an indispensable tool in medical and biological laboratories for a variety of applications. The PCR techniques involve the following basic ingredients: 1. The 4 nucleotide building blocks (dATP, dTTP, dCTP and d GTP); 2. A DNA polymerase (a heat stable enzyme derived from a thermophilic bacterium); 3. Two short oligonucleotides that serve as primers; 4. Target DNA of interest; 5. A buffer solution which provides a suitable chemical environment for optimum activity and stability of the DNA polymerase; 6. Divalent cation, magnesium or manganese ions; and 7. Monovalent cation potassium ions. The methods (Figure 4) depend on a thermal cycling consisting of an initial heating of up to 95^0C which causes the complementary strands of the target DNA to separate. When the mixture is cooled, the short oligonucleotide primers (~20bp long) find the complementary sites on the separate strands, then bind and provide the starting points for the DNA polymerase. These primers are attached to the flank of the region of the DNA to be synthesized. Adjusting to a third temperature allows for optimal DNA polymerase activity and the extension of the sequence for the two primers, which becomes a copy of the specific region of interest between the primers. The repeating of the cycle of heating and cooling leads to exponential growth in the number of DNA copies. A run of 30 cycles lasting only a few minutes and is sufficient to produce millions of identical copies of the target sequence of interest with the newly synthesized strands ranging from a few hundred base pair to several thousand.

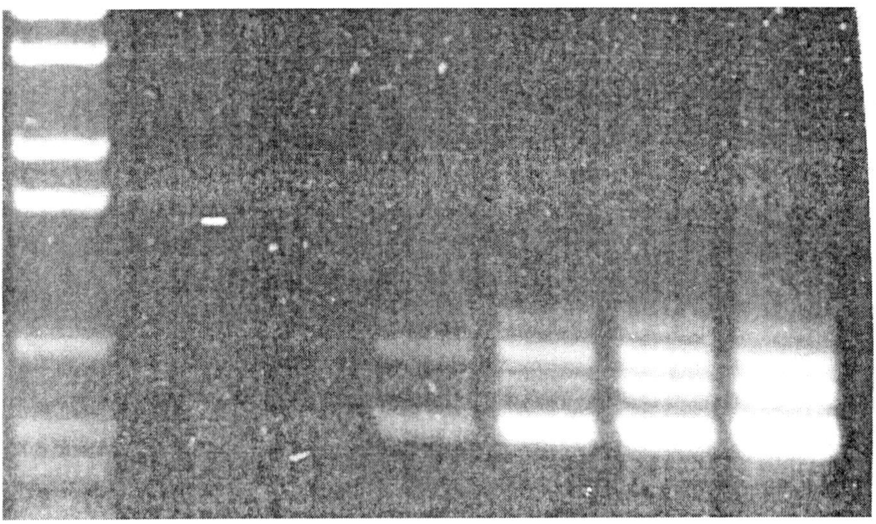

Figure 3. A typical PCR band. (Source: AHRO Laboratory)

To check whether the PCR procedure has generated the required DNA fragment (amplicon), agarose gel electrophoresis is used to separate the PCR products based on their sizes (Figure 3).

PCR can be used as an alternative method of malaria diagnosis because it allows for sensitive and specific detection of *Plasmodium* species DNA from the peripheral blood specimen. The PCR techniques may be more sensitive than conventional microscopy in very low parasitemias and more specific for species identification. PCR is also the best methodology for identifying key mutations in drug resistance. Table 3 below shows some of the uses of PCR in the malaria study.

Table 3. Application of simple PCR techniques to the epidemiological study of malaria parasite

1) Detection of sub patent infection
2) Detection of mixed infection
3) Study of the multiplicity of infections and their consequences
4) Search for virulence factors
5) Differentiation of recrudescence and reinfection after treatment
6) Detection of drug resistance markers

Use of Molecular Technique for Malaria Parasite Detection

Microscopy has been the “golden” technique for the primary detection of the malaria parasite as well as for species identification. However, this has some disadvantages since in most cases the morphology of the parasite is the main criteria used. The use of the DNA technique for the identification of the malaria parasite in the peripheral blood sample is now more reliable. This significantly improves the possibilities for the diagnosis and epidemiology of malaria. For example, a study has shown that *P ovale* consist of two major clades that diverged as different species. This finding was based on three different species such as the asexual stage expressed by the small subunit 18s rRNA, a nuclear gene encoding a cystein protease and mitochondrial *cytb* gene. The two major forms are not distinguishable morphological-wise. This means, that when studying the epidemiology of *P ovales*, it would be relevant to consider each separately using molecular techniques. Another finding that highlights the significance of molecular identification was a report from Southeast Asia. Due to the decline in the incidence of *P falciparum* and *P vivax* in the region, a large number of cases were surprisingly reported. This was initially considered to be due to *P malaria*e remaining in the Malaysian portion of Bornea. However, molecular phylogenetic and epidemiological studies showed that it was mostly due to the *P knowlesi*. More than a hundred cases were detected in the Kapit District of Sarawak over a 2-year period. During this period, no *P malariae* was detected by PCR. The *csp* gene of eight of the isolates is compared to *P knowlesi* from monkey and other malaria parasite species in a phylogenetic analysis. They were all indistinguishable from *P knowlesi* and showed some level of nucleotide polymorphism which suggested that they did not emerge recently from a single clonal source. A description of the uses of molecular techniques in malaria infection is discussed below.

Sub Patent Infection

Highly sensitive PCR techniques have been developed with the capacity of detecting parasites at a low density of 1 per microlitre or less. This is in contrast to the microscopic techniques where a threshold of about 10-50 parasites per microlitre is required for detection. In a study, the application of a sensitive PCR technique on blood samples which were obtained from children in an endemic area was positive almost every time. An examination of sequential samples has shown that parasitemia changes from day to day periodically until it reaches a level that can be detected by microscopy. This was found in a study by Van den Eede et al. who reported on a *P vivax* sub-patent infection in 3 patients which was followed by patent infection the following month. PCR analyses have shown that a complex pattern of malaria infection of different genotypes may occur in an individual who does not show any clinical signs of the infection.

Mixed Infection

In terms of epidemiological factors, the first question to be asked when using molecular techniques is what are the effects of a co-infection with one malaria parasite? For example, what is the effect of *P vivax* on *P falciparum*? Would it modify the course of infection? A study in Vanuatu showed that *P vivax* infection influences the severity of *P falciparum* malaria. In Thailand, co-infection wit*h P vivax* is associated with a reduction in the number of genotypes among Koren patients infected with *P falciparum*. In another PCR study in Cote d'Ivoire, it was shown that *P malariae* infection may reduce the risk of symptomatic *P falciparum* infection. The development of species-specific PCR techniques facilitated these types of studies.

Differentiate Recrudescence from Reinfection

Treatment failure is normally associated with drug resistance which may occur in areas where incidence of infection is low. However, in areas were individuals are bitten nearly every night by infected mosquitoes, the presence of the parasite indicated new infections. In the past, it was not possible to differentiate reinfection from recrudescence. Due to molecular techniques, this can now be done. The following has been suggested: If the parasite is present on follow-up at 2 or 3 loci to the parasite found on presentation then it is assumed that the infection is recrudescence. If the parasites are genetically different it is assumed that they indicate a new infection. This assumption is possibly valid but a number of contradicting factors have been identified. For example, if there are only a few parasitic genotypes circulating in a community as may be the case in areas of low transmission, then a new infection is likely to occur with a genetically identical parasite to the first. In addition, it is possible that the parasite detected at follow-up was present on presentation but at such a low density that even sensitive PCR techniques cannot detect them. Nevertheless, the technique is used in the evaluation of new antimalarial drugs and establishing rates of treatment failure. The antigens MSP1, MSP2 and GLURP are now widely used to differentiate recrudescence from reinfection.

Multiplicity Infection

Molecular analysis has shown that one individual can be simultaneously infected with multiple strains of the *Plasmodium* parasite that are genetically distinct, with such multiple strain infections believed to be associated with the development of strain-specific immunities. The number of genotypes found in individual infections varies from one to more than 10, depending on the gene that is used as the marker of multiplicity. Several studies have shown that there is a reduction with an increase in age in the number of genotypes present in infected individuals which suggests that it is due to acquired immunity. However, individuals may develop immunity to infection for some but not all strains to which they are exposed. In a study in Kenya, it was found that the multiplicity of infection increases with decreasing age with the changes more marked below 2 years. However, another study found that there was no such relationship, although the study was restricted to children below 5 years, meaning that we cannot rule out there can be some differences in older children.

Co-infection

One of the problems in the control of infectious diseases is the issue of co-infection. In the past, it was poorly understood due to the lack of proper diagnostic tools. Most of the available techniques such Giemsa- stain peripheral blood films are often tedious and labor intensive which requires expert intervention. To overcome this problem, the use of immune-chromatographic tests was suggested. The PCR technique has recently been known to be more sensitive and is being used for detecting co-infection in both epidemiological and clinical settings. Co-infection between *Plasmodium* and *Wuchereria bancrofti* is one of the public health problems currently plaguing tropical medicine. Two PCR-based assays have been developed for detecting *W bancrofti* and *Plasmodium* species. One is a real-time multiplex quantitative PCR that simultaneously detects *W bancrofti*, *P falciparum* and *P vivax* in mosquitoes. This can be extended to human malaria infection. This assay has been found to have a higher sensitivity than the conventional PCR assay thereby allowing for detecting initial parasite DNA at lower levels. The other is a multiplex assay which uses a set of four primers that amplify a 208bp fragment and a 450bp fragment of *W bancrofti* and a 208bp of *P falciparum.* Malaria and tuberculosis are endemic in many regions across the globe. A co-infection episode is one of the most interesting phenomena in infectious disease medicine. The advent of molecular techniques such bioinformatics will be of significant help in understanding the co-infection episode of malaria and TB.

Other co-infections of interest which have been exploited using molecular techniques are malaria and Africa Trypanosomiasis, malaria and HIV, malaria and dengue fever. To fill the gap in our understanding of co-infection episodes, there is the urgent need to study the co-infection of malaria and other conditions such as diabetes, hypertension and cancer which are now common in the tropics.

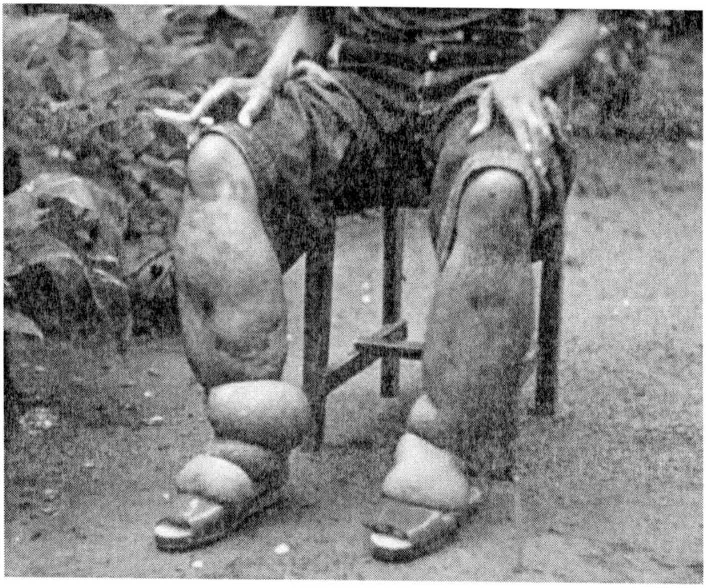

Figure 4. Elephantiasis due to *Wuchereria Broncrofti.* A co-infection with malaria can be traumatic. (Credit: CDC)

Current Picture

The World Health Organization reported that between 300 million and 500 million people are infected with malaria every year and that the disease is a public health problem in more than 90 countries 2.4 billion people, constituting about 40% of the global population. Sub-Saharan Africa is home to about 90% of all malaria cases and the remaining two-thirds are found in Afghanistan, Brazil, Colombia, India, Sri Lanka and Vietnam.

Distribution

P vivax and *P malariae* are globally distributed. Since ancient times, they have been characterized as "benign tertian" *(P vivax)* and "quartan" (*P malariae*) periodic fevers. "Benign tertian" was so named because they do not lead to severe and fatal manifestations of the "sub tertian" malignant periodic fever *(P falciparum*). Tertian and quartan are often referred to as those characteristic features of an acute episode that returns every third (*P vivax*) or fourth (*P malariae*) day. In the past, *P malariae* was the most dominant malaria parasite but it has now lost its dominance to *P vivax* and *P falciparum* which are now the most common malaria parasite encountered. *P vivax* is still found sporadically in some of the temperate regions of the world, which means reduction of *P vivax* malaria in those regions as it was widely prevalent in the past. It is, however, commonly prevalent in the tropics and subtropics. *P falciparum* is normally found in tropical, subtropical and warm temperate regions. This can be associated with the temperature limitation on its transmission by its vector. In the tropics, P *falciparum* remains the dominant malaria parasite and is widely prevalent. *P ovale* has a low risk fatal outcome and it is the most limited in terms of distribution. It is prevalent in Sub –Saharan Africa and is only endemic in the Philippines and New Guinea. Figure 5 shows the global transmission pattern of malaria.

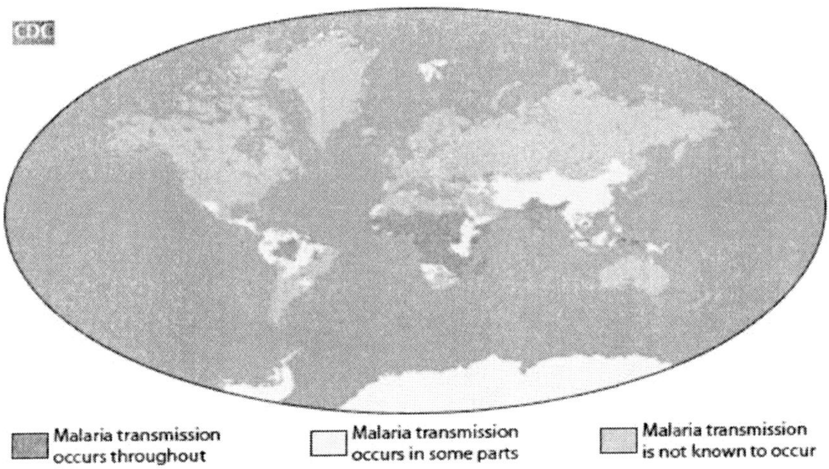

Figure 5. Global occurrence of malaria. (Credit: CDC)

Mortality Pattern

Malaria remains a threat to mankind in terms of morbidity, mortality and impact on economic growth. According to an estimate of the World Malaria Report 2010, about 781,000 malaria-associated deaths were recorded in 2009, with more than 80% of these cases occurring in Sub-Saharan Africa (SSA) especially in remote rural areas where there is poor access to health services. Measuring malaria mortality in populations is a challenge because malaria transmission intensity varies geographically. Therefore, the distribution of hospital cases and subsequent mortality rates may also exhibit some variations. Studies have been conducted to analyze the mortality burden of malaria and its associated factors. A study by Kazembe et al. to analyze the spatial variation and risk factors associated with malaria hospitalization and in-hospital mortality in a pediatric ward from 2002 to 2003 found that the rate of malaria hospitalization and in-hospital mortality decreased with age. The case fatality rate was associated with distance, age and wet season. It also increased if the patient was referred to the hospital. In addition, the death rate was high on the first day, followed by a relatively short stay in the hospital. Most of the studies on malaria mortality have been carried out in children. A descriptive retrospective study by Ngomane and de Jager in Mpumalange Province of South Africa found that malaria-associated mortality was lower in infants and children but higher in those over 65 years of age. They also found that the transmission pattern was related to the rainfall pattern. It has been shown that there is some degree of association between a high concentration of cases and malaria associated mortality but this is not absolute. Genetic variations among isolates of *P falciparum* have been shown to account for some foci of mortality. Virulent strains have also been mentioned. A study in Ghana found that young children and pregnant women were at the highest risk with respect to malaria morbidity and mortality with children under the age of 5 years the most vulnerable group. It was further shown that there is a distinction between the mortality patterns that peaked among children less than 5 years of age who accounted for 48.2% of total malaria deaths.

Another study involving seven demographic surveillance sites in areas across Sub-Saharan Africa with known stable endemics of *P falciparum* aimed at estimating the proportion of deaths by age group (3 month age groups up to 2 years of age and single year age group up to 15 years of age) using verbal autopsies (VAs), found that in all the sites, a substantial proportion of mortality which ranged from 20.1% in a Mozambican site to 46.2% in a site in Burkina Faso were attributed to malaria. On age pattern, it was similar in the different sites with deaths in the youngest children (under 3 months old) rarely linked to malaria. In children over 1 year old, the proportions of death associated with malaria were weakly dependent. In addition in most of the sites, all cause-deaths peaked during the rainy season but the strong seasonality in malaria transmission in these sites was not linked to strong seasonality in the number of deaths associated with malaria except in seven sites in Burkina Faso.

Maternal mortality is a major health problem. There has been series of studies conducted to estimate maternal mortality associated with malaria. There was a study in Maputo Mozambique to evaluate the impact of malaria associated maternal mortality by analyzing the seasonal variations of crude and malaria-specific maternal mortality rates between January 2001 and December 2003 by retrospectively checking the records. It found that during this period 278 deaths were recorded in which malaria was the most frequent cause of maternal deaths, accounting for 23%. The mortality rates showed similar patterns of seasonal variation peaking at the beginning and end of the malaria transmission season. The malaria associated mortality rate was found to be significantly higher during the rainy season. Similar results were confirmed in studies conducted in areas with similar transmission patterns in Senegal and the Gambia which showed that there was a significant increase in maternal mortality during the rainy seasons when it is known that malaria transmission is higher. However, there is no significant contribution of malaria as having a direct association with mortality. Therefore, malaria as a possible indirect cause of mortality was proposed.

Chapter IV

Pathogenesis and Clinical Features of Malaria Infection

Introduction

To understand the pathogenesis of human malaria infection, there is the need to investigate various mechanisms involving parasite invasion and host defense. The pathogenesis of a disease involves the various host and parasite factors that are responsible for causing the pathology. In this section, a review is made of the various factors related to the pathogenesis of human malaria infections.

Malaria Parasite and Human Immune System

Malaria infection induces a host response which is regulated by both innate and adaptive immunities. In defining malaria immunity, Bruce-Chwatt stated:" Malaria immunity may be defined as the state of resistance to the infection brought about by all those processes which are involved in destroying the plasmodia or by limiting their multiplication". Innate immunity, which is natural, is the inherent ability of the host, a refractory state or an immediate response which is inhibitory and due to the introduction of the parasite into the host. It is not dependent on past experience with the infection. Adaptive immunity, on the other hand, is acquired and may be either active or passive. Active immunity is due to the enhancement of the defense mechanism of the host due to a previous encounter with the parasite or even part of it. Passive immunity is due to immunity as a result of prenatal or postnatal transfer of a protective substance from mother to child or by introducing such a substance through injection as in vaccination.

The innate immune mechanism has been associated with low parasitaemia seen in acute *P falciparum*. The humoral and cellular mechanisms of the innate arm of the immune system are poorly defined but studies using a nonparasitic model have shown that a family of germ line encoded receptor proteins is highly significant for the innate immune mechanism for both invertebrates and vertebrates. In mammals, it has been shown that activation of macrophage through toll-like-receptor leads to the induction of effector genes which have the capability of controlling and executing the innate defense that is found in a large variety of bacterial and viral systems. This has not been investigated using parasitic models but it is believed that this system might be important for the innate defense against human malaria infections.

As a result of a malaria infection, there is usually an elevated concentration of non-malaria-specific immunoglobin. Neutrophils, mononuclear phagocytes and natural killer (NK) cells seem to have a role in innate immunity seen in early malaria infection. NK cells, in particular, have been shown to increase in number and lyse the *P falciparum*-infected erythrocyte. In addition, NK cells are potent producers of cytokines such as interferon-γ and therefore have a role in the activation of macrophage which plays an important function in malaria innate immunity as they have the potential of lysing infected host erythrocytes. Other cells which might have roles in innate malaria immunity are NKT cells, which in mice possess both NK1.1 surface markers and αβ T-cells receptors (TCR). These cells have been described as potent inhibitors of liver-stage parasite replication in mouse malaria model in vitro. Furthermore, NK1.1+ CD4+ murine T cells have been found to regulate Ig G antibody response to glycosylphosphatidyl inositol anchored *P falciparum* protein. This response might be important for a specific and rapid major histocompatibility complex (MHC) for unrestricted parasite control. T cells which are a γδTCR are expanded during the early stage of malaria infection and might have a role in innate parasite control. γδ T cells but not αβ T cells from malaria-naïve donors have been found to inhibit parasite replication in vitro. An explanation for this difference is linked to the difference in antigen recognition by the two types of TCR or even to the presence of γδ T cells of NK receptors, a non-antigen –specific ligation which results in rapid secretion of proinflammatory cytokines. In endemic areas, malaria infection results in strong humoral immune response which involves the production of Ig M and Ig G as well as other immunoglobin isotypes. A large proportion of this immunoglobin has been found to be non-malaria specific, reflecting the activation of polyclonal B-cell, about 5% or more of this represent species and stage- specific antigens reacting with a wide variety of the parasite antigen. Passive transfer of Ig G from immune donors leads to the reduction of parasite density and clinical disease. The innate immune system does not confer a long lasting protection but relies on the recognition of pathogen-associated molecular patterns (PAMPS). Following the recognition of the PAMPS, cell mediated response is induced which results in the elimination of the pathogen. In vertebrates, these responses involve inflammation and the recruitment of specialized cells to the site of infection through the production of effector molecules such as cytokine.

In humans, three types of acquired or adaptive immunity have been identified: A. anti-disease immunity which confers immunity against clinical disease and affects the risk and the level of morbidity associated with a given parasite density, B. antiparasite immunity which confers protection against the parasite affecting the density of the parasite and C. premonition which provides protection against new infections thereby maintaining low grade parasitemia and a general asymptomatic condition. Natural acquired immunity (NAI) to falciparum malaria provides protection for people across Sub-Saharan Africa where the disease is holoendemic. These people are almost continuously being infected with *P falciparum*. Adults have NAI but infants and young children occasionally do not possess NAI. NAI had been found to be compromised in pregnant women especially in primigravidae. Adults who have not been exposed to routine infections lose their NAI albeit temporarily. This means any intervention that reduces the risk of exposure below a certain threshold of maintaining NAI has the potential of creating a relapse as experienced in the highlands of Madagascar in the 1980s which resulted in a malaria epidemic that caused the death of more than 40,000 people. In addition, routine exposure to hyper- to holoendemic malaria provides protection to the majority of people while causing mortality among the minority. This means aggressive intervention that only considers the vulnerable minority risk compromising the protection against severe malaria among the majority. NAI provides protection against severe morbidity and mortality. Adults and older children in areas of hyper-to holoendemicity rarely experience life threatening complications associated with malaria.

HLA System and Malaria

The Human Leukocyte antigen (HLA) was discovered in the 1970s. The classical HLA loci are the Class I (HLA-A,-B,-C,-E) and Class II (HLA –DR,-DQ,-DM and –DP) molecules which were identified based on their role in antigen presentation to CD8+ and CD4+ T cells. They are encoded by a 4Mb region of human chromosome 6p21, recognized as the most variable region in the human genome. It is also designated as the major histocompatibility complex (MHC) due to the important role played by the Class I and Class II molecules in the recognition of self vs. nonself. Genes found in the MHC are known to play significant roles in transplant immunity and susceptibility to a wide range of diseases such as autoimmune and infectious diseases. Due to the role in presenting antigens to T-cells, these molecules are termed as the effectors and memorizers of acquired T-cell immunity.

Class I molecules are also recognized by Killer cell immunoglobulin-like receptor (KIR) molecules found on the surface of NK cells. A total of seventeen KIR have so far been identified. KIR elicits an additional role for the classical HLA molecules by causing the innate immune response to progress. Linkage of KIR by Class I molecules is said to provide positive or negative signals to NK cells through immunoreceptor tyrosine-based activating motifs (ITAMS) or immunoreceptor tyrosine-based inhibitory motifs (ITIM) found with KIR molecules. HLA and KIR are found on different chromosomes and are highly polymorphic. It has been argued that there is the potential for some combination between Class I and KIR alleles which can result in either beneficial or deleterious interactions. Such gene-gene interactions are known as epitasis. It has been found that other genes such as complement factors C2 and C4B, tumor necrosis factor (TNF) and lymphotoxin-α, are found in MHC. These genes regulate some aspect of the innate immune system. Based on this finding, the MHC is divided into Class I, Class III and Class II regions (Figure 7A) which show a movement from telomere to centriomere on 6p21. Sequence analysis across eight different homozygous MHC haplotypes has identified >44,000 variations both single-nucleotide polymorphisms (SNPs) and insertion deletion (indels) as well confirming the presence of >300 loci which include >160 protein-coding genes. The highly polymorphic regions are found in Class I and Class II genes.

Data available has shown that HLA loci are important genetic determinants of immune reaction to malaria infection. Various researchers have shown a connection between HLA Class II alleles and acquisition of antibodies to B-cell epitopes in the *P falciparum* ring-infected erythrocyte surface antigen (RESA), P126 antigen, glutamate-rich protein (GLURP) and repeated region of *P vivax* CSP. The African population possesses the largest genetic diversity within the HLA system'. For example, within Class I loci alone, extensive allelic diversity has been identified as follows: more than 600 HLA-A, 1100 HLA-B and 400

HLA-C alleles which are defined by variation at the protein sequence level. The Dogon tribes in Mali are examples of unique ethnic groups in Africa with high allelic diversity and genetic distance from the ancestral African population such as the Luo population of Kenya. It has been argued that this genetic diversity might pose some challenges in the development of a malaria vaccine which is aimed at developing cell-mediated immunity. HLA haplotypes were indirectly shown to elicit protection against natural infection through an association of HLA-B53 and the HLA class II block DRB1* 13:02-DQB1* 05:01 and protection against severe malaria in West Africa. Cytotoxic T-cell response to conserved epitopes of liver stage antigen (LSA)-1 and 3 which is restricted by class I allele B53 showed that T-helper cell response to the epitopes within CSP and LSA-1 elicit some protection against severe malaria, malaria-associated anemia and episodes of reinfection. In addition, genetic variations can also result in predisposition to variations of malarial disease such as cerebral malaria and severe malaria. It is possible that interferon-γ and interleukin-10 maybe associated with specific HLA polymorphism after rubella vaccinations.

Malaria severity and the subsets of malarial disease have been found to show discrete cytokine secretion patterns. A study by Lyke et al. to define the association of defined HLA alleles and the clinical outcome of malaria among children in northeast Mali established an association between HLA polymorphism and IL-10 production in severe malaria. They further found evidence of a possible correlation between two class I HLA alleles, A*30:01 and A*33:01 and the development of cerebral disease in Dogon children. Diakite et al. found that HLA-B associated transcript 2 (BAT2)-rs1046089 polymorphism maybe associated with severe malaria in the Gambian population. The BAT2 gene has been found to have microsatellite repeats which are implicated in the age-at-onset of insulin-dependent diabetes mellitus (IDDM) and the involvement of the inflammatory process of pancreatic β-cells destruction during the development of IDDM. The inflammatory role of BAT2 makes it an interesting issue in malaria research because of the important balance between inflammatory response induction against infection and inflammo-pathology which appears to be important in severe disease progression.

Other case-control studies have reported on the malaria/HLA association. A study of severe malaria in children in The Gambia found that HLA-B*5301 and HLA-DRB1*1302 were independently associated with resistance to severe malaria while in Western Kenya, an association between HLA-DRB1*0101 and resistance to severe malaria was also reported. Another study of severe malaria in children in Gabon found an association between DRB1*04 and DBP1*1701 and severe malaria. However, HLA-DQB1*0501 was associated with a decreased risk of reinfection and anemia. A study by Osafo-Addo et al. found that HLA-DRB1*04 might be significantly associated with susceptibility to severe malaria in the population in Northern Ghana. Association of DRB1*04 to severe malaria was independent of ethnic background. HLA-DRB1*04 is less common in the human population in Sub-Saharan Africa than in the population of the rest of the world. This is consistent with a strong negative selection by endemic *P falciparum* malaria.

The HLA-KIR receptor-ligand combinations have been hypothesized to be associated with cerebral malaria and that KIR and HLA ligand diversity has been shaped by fatal malaria as selective pressure in malaria endemic areas. Hirayasu et al. found that the KIR2DL3-HLAC1 receptor-ligand is significantly associated with the development of cerebral malaria in Thailand. Furthermore, comparison of both the KIR2DL3 and the HLA-C1 gene frequencies between malaria and high-endemic and non-endemic populations suggests that natural selection has acted on both KIR2DL3 and HLA-C1.

Immune Evasion in Malaria Infection

The malaria parasite has evolved a mechanism to escape detection and subsequent destruction by the immune system. In *P falciparum* malaria it has been shown that epigenetic mechanisms are used in switching off the expression of the variant surface protein which is encoded by the virulence *(var)* gene family. In this way it is able to evade the host immune responses. The antibody IgM plays an important role in malaria pathogenesis as it has been shown that parasite-specific IgM limits the replication of parasites. Natural IgM binds to the surface of *P falciparum* infected erythrocytes via the Fc. This has been argued to correlate with severe malaria in laboratory strains. Furthermore, non immune IgM binding is only shown by a subset of *P falciparum* isolates but still linked to the most severe clinical effects of malaria. The binding of IgM to *P falciparum*-infected erythrocyte is via the parasite variant antigen *P falciparum* erythrocyte membrane protein one (PfEMP1) found on the surface of infected erythrocytes. The PfEMP1 variants are encoded by *var* genes and each parasite contains between 50-60 var genes in its genome; with only one variant expressed on the infected erythrocyte surface at a time. A study showed that var genes are switched by heterochromatin silencing. Because only one var gene is expressed at a time and the other genes are wrapped in dense transcriptionally inactive forms of chromatin, activation of a different var gene when the parasite has to evade the immune response involves moving the silenced chromatin into position in the nucleus that is permissive for expression. It was initially estimated that the switch rate in *P falciparum* could be as high as 2%. However, it is now clear that these rates change in different variants. Studies have shown that all *var* genes are capable of being expressed in situ in an exclusive manner. Earlier Deitsch et al. showed that silent var promoters became transcriptionally active when removed from the chromosome and placed on transfected episomes in *P falciparum.* Freitas-Junior et al. identified key epigenetic factors that control the expression of *var* genes which are crucial molecules in immune escape and pathogenesis of *P falciparum.* In their study, they discovered two distinct chromatin modifications that led to the silencing of the *var* genes. Heterochromatin (involving Sir2-like protein) was one modification that was propagated from the telomeres over more than 50kb into the chromosome-coding region. They also showed that epigenetic silencing of the *var* genes is a reversible process which is dependent on histone acetylation at promoter regions. This study proved that dynamic chromatin changes control antigenic variations in malaria parasites. There is the need for more studies to understand the molecular aspects of immune evasion in *P falciparum* malaria which could possibly result in the development of vaccine (will be discussed later).

Biomarkers of Virulence

Hulka and colleagues defined biomarkers as "cellular, biochemical or molecular alterations that are measureable in biological media such as human tissues, cells, or fluids". This definition has recently been expanded to include biological characteristics that can be measured and evaluated as an indicator of normal biological processes, pathogenic processes or pharmacological responses to therapeutic interventions. Biomarkers include the tools and techniques needed to understand the prediction, cause, diagnosis, progression, regression or outcome of the treatment of diseases. For malaria, there is an effort towards identifying biomarkers that can accurately discriminate the severe forms of malaria. The use of biomarkers in clinical practices requires a stringent validation of their utility. Pepe et al. proposed at least five plans of biomarker development for cancer which was recently adapted by Coca and Parikh for acute kidney injuries. In summary, the initial phase involves the development of a clinical assay (s) that is capable of measuring the potential biomarker. The assay must be able to detect the disease and validate the biomarkers. In the third phase, retrospective longitudinal studies are undertaken to test the new biomarkers for their utility. During this phase, the sensitivity and specificity should be determined. The fourth phase involves the prospective screening in which the identified biomarker is used to screen a large population to determine their utility. In the final phase, the biomarker is analyzed for its ability to have an impact on disease control and management. A successful biomarker should have a reasonable impact on disease management.

Why are biomarkers important in malaria management? It is known that the transition from mild malaria to severe malaria can be sudden. This requires immediate intervention. The use of biomarkers can be used to risk-stratify severe malaria patients which can go a long way to better patient care and assist in the proper management of health resources. Biomarkers can also identify asymptomatic cases that might be harboring large numbers of the parasites that go undetected with a light microscope or other conventional diagnostic methods. This will be crucial in monitoring the elimination of malaria reservoirs from endemic populations. It can therefore be argued that biomarkers for malaria management are essential and a necessity. There has been series of biomarkers proposed in malaria management. Studies by Jain et al. undertaken in Ghana and India showed a striking association between the chemokine interferon inducible protein (CXCL10) and the severity of CM. Thus, there is a suggestion that CXCL10 might be a biomarker for CM severity. A study by Witt et al. with the aim of evaluating the diagnostic accuracy of plasma Triggering Receptor Expressed on Myeloid Cell 1 (TREM-1), neopterin and procalcitonin levels as biomarkers of severe *P falciparum* disease among 104 travelers with imported malaria found that there were no significant differences in TREM-1 levels between the different patient groups. However, patients with severe *P falciparum* had significantly higher levels of neopterin and procalcitonin when compared to patients with uncomplicated *P falciparum* or no *P falciparum* malaria. The authors concluded that neopterin and procalcitonin can be used as biomarkers for the rapid exclusion of severe malaria diseases on admission although their diagnostic value is limited.

Conroy et al., in their study tested the hypothesis that endothelium-derived biomarkers are associated with the pathophysiology of severe malaria and that it might be used in identifying children with CM, suggested that the endothelial proteins can be used as biomarkers of severe malaria disease. When it comes to anemia in malaria infection, Ong'echa et al. attempted to identify the strongest biomarkers of anemia by using a parsimonious set of predictor variables for hemoglobin (Hb) which was generated by least angle regression (LAR) controlling for the confounding effects of age, gender, G6PD deficiency and sickle cell traits followed by multiple linear regression analysis reported that IL-12p70 and IFN-$_\gamma$ emerged as positive predictors of Hb while IL-2R, IL-13 and eotaxin were negatively associated with Hb. They, therefore, concluded that IL-12p70/IFN-$_\gamma$ pathway represents a set of biomarkers that predict elevated levels of Hb in children with falciparum malaria while activation of the IL-13/eotaxin pathway favors anemia. Others have also recommended the use of changes in surface morphologies such as surface lesions and furrow-like structures as biomarkers for malaria diagnosis in addition to elevated stiffness and cytoadhesion characteristics.

To identify hepatic compromise, there is the recommendation that changes in liver function markers such as aminotransferase (AST), alanine aminotransferase (ALT), alkaline phosphatase (ALP) activities and bilirubin (total, conjugated and unconjugated) can be important. Management of severe malaria using biomarkers will require three main categories of biomarkers: early biomarkers, diagnostic biomarkers and prognostic biomarkers. However, the development of biomarkers is a long journey which will require some technological tools. After the validation of the biomarkers, the format for the identified biomarker needs to be formulated. To introduce biomarkers within the clinical setting, one challenge to be faced is the cost. Most malaria cases occur in resource limited settings. There is the concern of whether expensive detection methods can be used as practical tools. The recent development of simpler and more field appropriate tools should be a guide that reliable biomarkers can also be measured using simple methods. It is the hope of the author that such simple technology will be available for biomarkers when they become available.

Clinical Manifestations

Infection with *Plasmodium falciparum* can lead to a series of different clinical manifestations in humans ranging from no symptoms to mild flu-like symptoms to coma and death. The classic clinical presentation associated with malaria consists of bouts of fever, accompanied by other symptoms such as chills, sweating, headache, malaise, nausea, muscular pains, anemia, jaundice, swelling of the spleen and mild bouts of diarrhea. Individuals with mild or uncomplicated malaria do not generally present any features of severe or complicated malaria (Table 4). Severe manifestations of malaria include cerebral malaria, liver dysfunction, acute kidney injury, bleeding, acute respiratory distress syndrome, severe malarial anemia (SME, hemoglobin (HB) <5.0g/dl), hypoglycemia, hyerlactatemia and multiple organ failures. Some of these are briefly dealt with below.

Table 4. WHO Criteria of Severe Malaria

• A score on the Glasgow Come Scale of less than 11 (indicating CM)
• Anemia (hematocrit <20%) with parasite counts exceeding 100,000 µl (roughly corresponding to 2% parasitemia on peripheral blood smear)
• Jaundice (serum bilirubin >50µmol/l) with parasite counts exceeding 100,000/µl on peripheral blood smear.
• Renal impairment /urine output (400ml/24h and serum creatinine >250µmol/l.
• Hypoglycemia (blood glucose <2.2mmol/l
• Hyperparasitaemia (>10% parasitemia
• Systolic blood pressure <80mmHg with cold extremities

Human Cerebral Malaria

The most severe complication associated with *Plasmodium falciparum* is cerebral malaria (CM) which is clinically defined by the World Health Organization (WHO) to include the following: a Blantyre coma score of <2, *P falciparum* parasitemia by blood film and no evident cause of coma such as meningitis or hypoglycemia. The most definitive diagnosis of CM relies on post-mortem examination of the brain either by autopsy or through supraorbital sampling. The finding of malarial retinopathy on ophthalmoscope in comatose patients has been argued to be a yardstick of CM. CM is known as the most common clinical presentation and cause of death in severe malaria yet the mechanism of pathogenesis and what causes death in fatal cases is still poorly understood. However, different hypotheses have been suggested. It has been postulated that an essential feature of severe falciparum malaria is sequestration of the erythrocyte which is found to contain a mature form of the parasite in deep vascular beds. Sequestration is greatest in the brain. This may explain the rationale why coma is a prominent feature in CM. The reason behind the sequestration of the parasite is unknown but it is believed that they grow better in an oxygen-depleted environment than in ambient air and binding to the endothelium is one method of circumventing spleen-associated destruction. CM is fatal if left untreated and is associated with an 80% fatality in treated patients. The WHO proposed three pathogenic theories for human CM:

a) The immunological theory: This states that the neuropathological findings in human CM can be linked to hyperergic reactions of the central nervous system to antigenic challenges as a result of infection by *P falciparum*. It has been argued that epidemiological data suggests that cerebral lesion in man could be attributed to immunopathological reactions. The complication is frequently found in children and non-immune individuals. The immunological connections are further supported by data which showed a lower incidence in malnourished children from endemic areas that had deficient cell-mediated immunity. Decreased cell-mediated immune response can be associated with a decreased prevalence of CM.
b) Permeability Theory: This originated from the findings which showed that increased blood-brain barrier permeability to ^{125}I-labeled albumins to a *P knowlesi*-infected rhesus monkey; with the suggestion that it might be mediated by kinins.
c) Mechanical Theory: This states that "pathophysiology of severe *falciparum* malaria might be explained by microcirculation obstruction with consequent local hypoxia and ischemia".

Several factors have been hypothesized to have a role in the pathogenesis of CM. A study by Milner et al. using a molecular assay implicated genetic complexity in CM and suggested that single / low complexity infections are more likely to lead to death. Over production of cytokine was detected in an experimental CM which was implicated in brain vascular pathology. A study reported that gamma-interferon is an important mediator in the pathogenesis of CM. It has also been shown that helper T lymphocytes play a role in the development of CM in murine while cytokine-induced phenotypic changes in the brain microvascular endothelial cells (MVEC) play key roles in the sequestration event in both parasitized blood cells and parasitized leukocytes. TNF has been identified as key mediators in experimental CM as studies have shown high levels of TNF in serum during CM, prevention of neurological syndrome through in vivo neutralization TNF and induction of CM-like syndrome in CM-resistant mice through infusion of TNF. Recently, it has been found that transgenic mice expressed high levels of TNF receptor 1 (TNFR1) and in TNF/LT gene knockout mice. This proves that TNF had a role in CM. Clinical studies also showed that the anti-TNF monoclonal antibody (Mab) in humans leads to a significant reduction in malaria fever. This implies that TNF play a role. Furthermore, there is a hypothesis which states that regulation of platelet -decorated ULVWF (ultra-large von Willebrand factor) plasma protease ADAMTS13 (a distrigin and metalloproteinase with a thrombospondin type 1 motif, member 3) may have a role in CM development with some studies supporting this hypothesis. Significant reduction of plasma ADAMTS13 function was seen in cerebral or severe malaria patients in comparison to healthy subjects. A study by Kraisin et al. found that single nucleotide polymorphism (SNP) of ADAMTS13, rs4962153 was found to be associated with cerebral malaria in 708 Thai patients with *P falciparum* malaria. Changes in cerebral microvasculature such as petechial hemorrhage, breakdown of the blood-brain barrier, edema and congestion have been reported in later stages of murine CM. Cerebral microvasculature has long been recognized to be the main manifestation in the pathology of CM. Human cerebral malaria (HCM) occurs normally 2 weeks after the mosquito bite and may develop 2 to 7 days later. Seizures, retinopathy and brainstem alteration as a result of elevated intracranial pressure and brain swelling, are common clinical features of HCM. Neurological symptoms are associated with anemia, severe metabolic acidosis and hypoglycemia. Patients with HCM usually die quickly before the commencement of therapy and patients who survive it may develop long-term neurological sequelae, cognitive and behavioral deficits.

Placental Malaria

In Sub-Saharan Africa, about 32 million pregnant women are reported to be at risk of infection by *P falciparum*. Only a handful of infections have been noted in pregnancy. Maternal mortality associated with *P falciparum* malaria is highest in areas of low and unstable transmission or in epidemic, whereas in higher transmission, the main complications of *P falciparum* during pregnancy are maternal anemia and low birth weight which has been estimated to result in 100,000 infants death in Africa. These effects are normally most severe in primigravidae but also in areas of low transmission, women of higher gravidity are mostly affected.

In *P vivax* infection, placenta malaria (PM) is also associated with maternal anemia and low birth weight. However, the anemia caused by *P vivax* is less severe than that caused by *P falciparum*. *P falciparum* sequesters in the placenta which leads to fetal damage through interference with fetomaternal nutrient exchange and some local immunological changes which results in the secretion of type 1 cytokines. Cytoadherance which emanates from sequestration may be compounded by resetting and agglutination. Resetting is known to occur in *P vivax*. It has been reported that women who were parasiteamic once during their pregnancy deliver low birth weight children. This means that either *P vivax* sequesters for a long time in the placenta or is able to relapse at undetectable concentration or sequestration of the parasite in the placenta. It is one of the major causes of adverse impact on the uncomplicated *P falciparum* or *P vivax* malaria on the fetus. It has also been reported that maternal-fetal immunological interaction type 2 cytokine are believed to protect the fetus. *P vivax* can induce a shift towards a type-1 response resulting in similar consequences like those in *P falciparum* infection which raises the concentration of type 1 proinflammatory cytokines in the placenta resulting in lower birth weight. A switch to T-helper response has been found to have an adverse impact on the placenta; fetus or both that persist long after parasitization. Intrauterine growth is affected by *Plasmodium* malaria. This growth retardation is associated with the accumulation of *P falciparum* infected red cells in the placenta. The accumulation is due to adherence to specific and relatively conserved cell surface expressed domain of the antigenically variant protein (PfEMP1) to the placental glucosaminoglycan chondroitin sulphate A and the secondary receptor like immunoglobulin and hyaluronic acid. In *P vivax* malaria, adherence of *P vivax*-infected erythrocyte to the glucosaminoglycan might have a role in the pathogenesis of vivax malaria which leads to the retardation of intrauterine growth.

A study found that excessive complement activation is essential in the pathogenesis of PM by mediating inflammation, coagulation and endothelial dysfunction. It further suggested that mutation in the mannose-binding lectin (MBL) and mannan-binding lectin serine peptidase 2 (MASP2) proteins might have a direct role on the susceptibility of PM. A great concern is the effect of HIV on placental malaria and vice versa. HIV-1 complicates the adverse consequences of PM by increasing the risk of infection, parasite densities and the severity of the disease. It also impairs response to antimalaria drug therapy. Increased risk of maternal anemia, maternal mortality; most frequent among the primigravidae and younger women as well as HIV infection are some of the manifestations associated with PM. A variety of adverse perinatal outcomes have been described, such as preterm delivery, intrauterine delivery and reduction in anthropometric parameters including: fetal anemia, congenital malaria and increased mother-to child transmission of HIV are all associated with PM. A study reported on PM-associated hypertension among young first-time mothers with histological features of chronic disease. Antimalaria prophylaxis can be used.

Severe Malarial Anemia (SMA)

The World Health Organization defines SMA as HB concentration of <5.0g/dl or a hematocrit of <15.0% in the presence of any density parasitemia. SMA is one of the major public health problems associated with malaria in developing countries where it is believed to contribute 3-46% of pediatric in-patient fatality cases. There has been a great amount of effort towards reducing the burden of SMA but it remains an important childhood health problem in Sub Saharan Africa. A study showed that SMA affects about 7.5-34% of Africa's children that acquire malaria with an overall estimate of 21.2% prevalence and case fatality of 8.4%. Several etiological factors have been associated with SMA. These include lysis of infected and uninfected RBCs, dyserythropoiesis, splenic sequestration, bone marrow suppression, co-infection with bacteriemia, HIV and hook worm as well as the chronic transmission of malaria in holoendemic areas. What causes low level Hb in SMA? Several mechanisms have been described in the pathogenic process of SMA. First, low levels of Hb in children with SMA are associated with impaired and / or ineffective erythropoiesis. This can be explained as follows: the loss of appropriate production of erythrocytes results in a failure to replenish the reduced pool of erythrocytes as a result of parasite- and / or anti-malaria-driven hemolysis.

Dormer et al. demonstrated that there is parenchyma damage of bone marrow, ineffective erythropoisis and a reduced rate of erythropoietic proliferation in patients with acute *falciparum* malaria resulting in low Hb while Were et al. also showed that taking into consideration the reticulocyte production index (RPI), children with SMA were characterized by levels <2.0. The RPI is defined as the measure of the extent to which the relationship with reticulocyte has risen or not in response to the level of anemia. All of these demonstrate that suppression of erythropoiesis is a primary cause of severe anemia in *falciparum* malaria in children. Others have linked inefficient eryhtopoiesis in SMA to an imbalance in inflammatory mediators and other studies linked it to hemozoin formation and inflammatory mediators such as interleukin (IL)-12, TNF and interferon (INF). There is the need to explore more to understand the pathogenic process that leads to the suppression of erythropoiesis. This will offer better treatment options to reduce the morbidity and mortality associated with SMA.

Black Water Fever

Black Water Fever (BWF) also referred to as malarial hemoglobinuria and "fievre bilieuse hemoglobinurique" (FBH) by French writers is defined as an entity which involves the combination of severe intravascular hemolysis, anemia, jaundice, hemoglobinuria and passage of black or red urine which may result in renal failure and death. Table 5 outlines some of the clinical findings in a hospital in Vietnam. Most of the cases are associated with *P falciparum* malaria with limited or often no parasitemia. In general, it was frequently found in the past in non-immune individuals who irregularly took quinine as a chemoprophylactic drug and were not treating *P falciparum* malaria adequately; although isolated cases has been associated with other antimalarial drugs such halofantrine and mefloquine. The introduction of chloroquine as a drug of choice for treating malaria resulted in a drop of BWF cases. G6PD has been implicated in BWF with the suggestion that its deficiency is frequently associated with BWF. This is not a determinant as BWF has also been described in patients with normal G6PD who were on quinine for severe malaria. The pathogenesis of BWF remains unclear but the role of quinine seems to be important although there has been an argument against this in that antibodies directed against quinine have never been detected in patients with BWF. In addition, a study by Wery et al. showed that of 28 cases of BWF, 25% had not taken quinine but from data gathered by Wery et al., it was concluded that BWF might be as a result of the relative inefficiency of quinine when used irregularly as a suppressor drug. Therefore the presumed triggering factors of BWF are halofantrine (38%), quinine (24%), mefloquine (24%) and halofantrine with quinine (14%)

Table 5. Clinical Manifestation associated with Blackwater fever (References Bodi et al., Gobbi et al. and Rivera et al.)

- Fever
- Rigor
- Severe anemia
- Severe intravascular hemolysis
- Dark urine
- Acute renal failure (ARF)
- Jaundice
- Hepatomegaly
- Splenomegaly
- Patient can be asymptomatic
- Low parasitemia

There is no agreed consensus regarding the antimalarial treatment regimen during BWF. However, the presumption is that the triggering agent should be withdrawn immediately. Nevertheless, antimalarial treatment is needed for patients who are parasitemia and or have preexisting tropical splenomegaly. Due to the chance of possible cross-reactivity between quinine, halofantrine and mefloquine, fansider, ACT and atovaquone-proguanil should be considered as additional drugs during treatment. After an episode of BWF, it is advisable to refrain from giving quinine, halofantrine and mefloquine because of the risk of recurrence. Therefore, other agents should be used as prophylaxis and curative treatment. The risk of BBWF should also be taken into consideration when quinine, halofantrine or mefloquine is administered for malaria in long-term expatriates to Africa.

Liver Dysfunction

Liver dysfunction has been recognized in malaria infection and injury to the liver is regarded as one of the most dreaded complications of severe malaria. However, some have disputed the clinical significance of this finding. It has been found that the involvement of the renal system varies from mild proteinuria to severe ozotomia associated with metabolic acidosis. Acute tubular necrosis (ATN) and mild proliferative glomurulonephropathy have been identified as the most common renal lesion associated with malaria. Jaundice has also been identified as having a close relationship between the incidence of severe malaria and liver damage. It has been postulated that jaundice is due to intravascular hemolysis of erythrocytes, hepatic dysfunction associated with hemoglobinopathies as well as microangiopathic haemolysis which is associated with intravascular coagulation. Jaundice has been reported more often in *falciparum* than *vivax* malaria as described by Hazra et al. who found jaundice in 40% and 9.09% cases of *P falciparum* and *P vivax* respectively. A study by Seth et al. also reported 7.7% cases of jaundice in *P falciparum* and non in *P vivax.* Most of the studies analyzing liver function and severe malaria reported of changes in biomarkers associated with the function of the liver. There has been a report of an increase in the mean activity of various liver enzymes as shown in a study in Nigeria (Table 4), serum (total) and unconjugated bilirubin. The WHO advises that a serum creatinine level above 265μmol/L is an indication of acute renal failure (ARF). A low and falling albumin level has been found to be important parameter of hepatic dysfunction. The WHO advised that clinical signs of liver failure such as liver flaps or asterixis are almost always seen concomitantly with viral hepatitis which highlights the role of co-infection in the pathogenesis of liver dysfunction.

The pathogenesis of hepatitis in malaria is unclear although there has been some excellent work on this topic. A study by Devarbhavi et al. involving 25 patients with fulminant hepatic failure in malaria found that in most of the cases, prothrombin time and liver span remained normal. This suggests that the liver's synthetic function is preserved. The abnormal liver biomarkers might be secondary to the release of various cytokines such as tumor necrosis factor (TNF). Hepatocyte necrosis has been reported absent or spotty in a series of studies. Hepatocyte dysfunction and cholestasis has been associated with impaired secretion of bile secondary to the loss of microvilli in bile canaliculi and the local disturbance of blood in the sinusoids. Histological examination has revealed hepatocyte necrosis, cholestasis, granulomatous lesions, bile stasis and focal accumulation, sinusoidal dilatation and congestion with hyperplasia of the Kupffer cell.

Can Automated Red Blood Cell (RBC) Be Used for Treating Severe *Plasmodium falciparum* Malaria?

Severe malaria caused by *P falciparum* is associated with high mortality despite the appropriate management techniques employed in intensive care units. Few interventions such as parenteral artesunate, mechanical ventilation and renal replacement have been found to be effective. However, other adjunctive treatments such as corticosteroids to reduce cerebral edema and anticonvulsive drugs in CM did not improve the patient's outcome. Some were even implicated in an increased rate of sequelae and deaths. Whole blood transfusion has been proposed as a method which can rapidly reduce parasite biomass. Riddle et al. in a meta-analysis of eight case-control studies involving 279 patients showed that whole blood exchange transfusion was not superior to antimalarial chemotherapy alone. This resulted in the discouraged use of this method. Automated RBC exchange might provide the answer that may potentially overcome problems associated with whole blood exchange. In this technique, RBCs are separated automatically from the whole blood of the patient. The plasma, platelets and white blood cells are retained. Various studies on different indications have shown that this procedure is better tolerated in comparison to whole blood exchange transfusion with regards to volume alteration, coagulation and electrolyte disturbances and susceptibility to infection. RBC exchange has been successfully used in patients with sickle cell crisis. It has therefore been advocated for use as adjunctive treatment potential for severe malaria. Some case reports have shown that automated RBC exchange has therapeutic potential in some patients. A study by Auer-Hackenberg et al. using RBC exchange as an adjunctive treatment for severe *falciparum* malaria in cohort patients treated at the Medical University of Vienna, Austria between 2000 and 2010 found that automated RBC exchange was a safe and efficient procedure which rapidly clears peripheral parasitaemia. It was well tolerated without any sign and symptom of clinical deterioration, electrolyte disturbances or bleeding complications. Despite exchanging about 1-1.5 times the volume of the patients total RBC pool, apheresis did not lead to problems of fluid overload and haemodynamic distress which are associated with whole blood exchange transfusion. Furthermore, during or shortly after automated RBC exchange, no specific medical intervention became necessary to maintain haemodynamic and respiratory stability. In a case report by Weir et al. involving three patients who were admitted with CM, they initiated antimalarial therapy immediately and an automated RBC exchange was done as an emergency measure. They found that the parasitaemia levels were less than 1% in all patients 24 hours after the last exchange. The neurologic status of the patients returned to baseline. They, therefore, concluded that an automated RBC exchange transfusion can rapidly reduce the level of parasitaemia and the neurologic functioning was resolved.

Automated RBC exchange has been found to be safe and can rapidly reduce parasitaemia in critical patients. However, quality data from randomized controlled studies are lacking. This makes it impossible to predict the risk-benefit ratio of this procedure for severe malaria. It has been shown that total biomass correlates with the severity of *falciparum* malaria but remains unclear whether physical removal of the parasite can improve a patient's outcome. It can, however, be postulated that rapid reduction of parasitaemia can have some profound benefit to the patients at a high risk for adverse outcome. This includes non-immune travelers and people living in regions with unstable malaria transmission patterns. Some have argued that the risk-benefit of this procedure depend on the antimalarial agent used and its speed of action.

Malaria Diagnosis

The simplest method of diagnosing malaria infection in the clinical setting has been the use of staining a patient's blood sample with Giemsa's, Wright's or Field's on a slide and then examining the slide microscopically (Figure 6). If the patient is actually infected, the plasmodia parasites become visible in the erythrocytes. This method, which is the "gold standard "for detecting malaria infection, is very effective in resource limited settings and is sensitive. However, this method is time consuming, labor intensive and requires high-quality microscopes and equipment, highly qualified personnel and due to detection limitation, it can delay the initiation of treatment. For example, this method cannot detect very low parasitemias. Another disadvantage of routine microscopy examination is mixed infection can be missed especially when the infection is caused by either P *malaria* or *P ovale*. Recently, new methods of detecting malaria infection have been introduced.

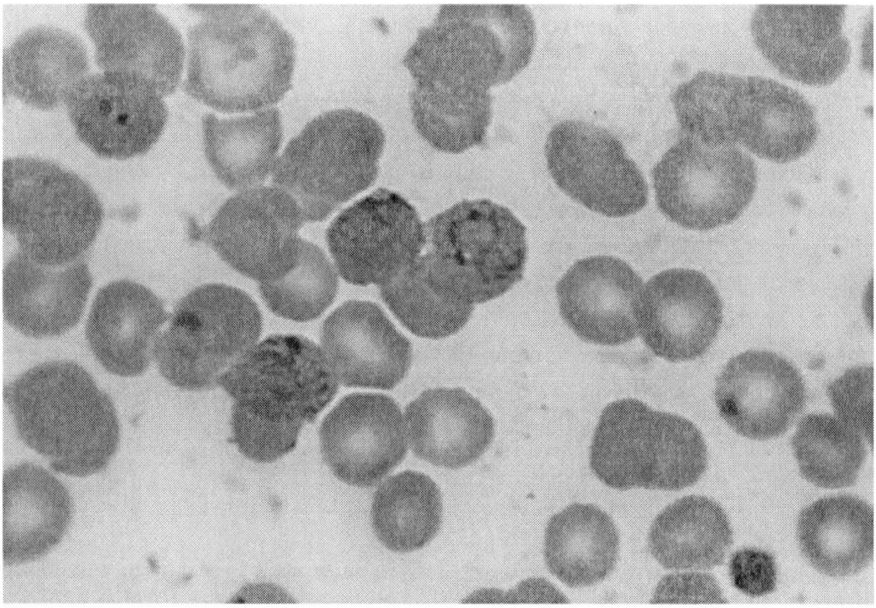

Figure 6. A micrograph depicting red blood cells infected by P falciparum. (Credit: CDC)

These methods include the use of tagged monoclonal antibodies to detect malaria antigens, flow cytometry, fluorescence microcopy, acridine orange staining, serology, molecular amplification techniques such as polymerase chain reactions (PCR), loop-mediated isothermal amplification (LAMP), automated analysis of blood cells, laser desorption mass spectrometry, buffer coat analysis, etc. These methods have their strengths and weaknesses. However, the need for specialized equipment, assay run time, operator expertise and cost can make its applicability in an acute infection setting very limited. The use of the rapid method for malaria detection is now recommended by the WHO. It is fast and easy to use and does not require electricity or complex equipment. In rapid diagnostic tests (RDTs), a patient's blood is applied to either a pad or plate which contains a specific malaria antigen. If visible bands show after a short time, then the patient has malaria. At its 2000 Congress, the World Health Organization outlined some recommendations on the use of RDTs. The conclusions drawn from the recommendations were: the results from this procedure should be as accurate as microscopy results performed by an average technician and the sensitivity should be above 95% when compared to microscopy. RDTs are now manufactured by about 60 companies. This continuous increase in the number of suppliers and their variables make it difficult for policy makers of national malaria programs to determine which tests are more suitable within their settings.

The RDT is based on the principle of lateral-flow immunochromatographic technology which is based on capturing the parasite antigen from peripheral blood using monoclonal or polyclonal antibodies that are prepared against a specific malaria antigen target which is then conjugated to a liposome in a mobile phase. It has been found that monoclonal antibodies can be more specific but less sensitive while polyclonal antibodies are more sensitive but less specific. Second or third monoclonal antibodies are sprayed to a strip of nitrocellular membrane which binds to the membrane in an immobile phase. When the antigen-antibody complex migrates (in the mobile phase) along the strip, the labeled antigen is captured by the monoclonal antibody in the immobile phase resulting in the production of a visible line if the target antigen is present in the test sample. The migration process depends on certain factors which include the porosity of membrane, the buffer used and the components of the reagents. Figure 7 shows the format of RDTs.

There are over 100 different brands available and most are based on the detection of either histidine-rich protein 2 (HRP2), a *P falciparum* synthesized protein, lactate dehydrogenase (LDH) or aldolase, two enzymes produced by all the human *Plasmodium* species. Studies have shown that HRP2 remain longer in circulation as LDH or aldolase after the successful treatment of malaria. This may increase the proportion of false positive results. It has, therefore, been recommended that the HRP2 based test may not be ideal for areas with high malaria transmission due to the incidence of repeated attacks. However, LDH disappears quickly after successful treatment.

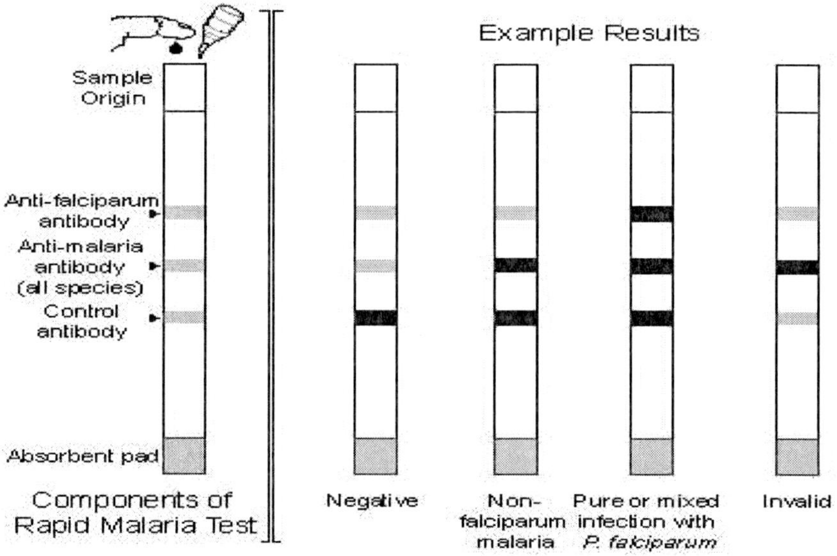

Figure 7. Diagrammatic representative of Malaria RDT format. (Adopted from Kakkilaya, 2003)

Examples of RDT Available

Optimal-IT®

This was developed by DiaMed Basel Switzerland which is LDH dependant and has been found to perform well in stable transmission areas. It has 98% sensitivity and 95% specificity. In a study by Tarimo et al., they concluded that optimal-IT® has an almost ideal accuracy.

Paracheck-pf®

It is a HRP2 RDT which was developed by Orchid Biomedical Services India. A study concluded that this test would be of immense benefit for *P falciparum* screening in areas that do not provide microscopy services but persistence of the HRP-2 antigen in the bloodstream after treatment can affect the interpretation of the result.

CareStart Malaria ^{Tm} (AccessBio Inc)

This three-band RDT detects Pf-pLDH and pan *Plasmodium* specific pLDH (pan-pLDH). A study concluded that this RDT maybe an alternative to other well-described HRP-2 three band RDTs in the non-endemic areas. Its performance for the detection of *P ovale* and *P malariae* is mediocre.

VIKIA Malaria Ag Pf/pan^{TM}

This test was developed by IMACCESS®, a company whose aim is to address public health needs by developing reliable diagnostic tests in response to the constraint associated with use in a field population in developing countries. The test is based on the same technology as other RDTs allowing for the detection of falciparum malaria (HRP-2) and non-falciparum malaria (aldolase).

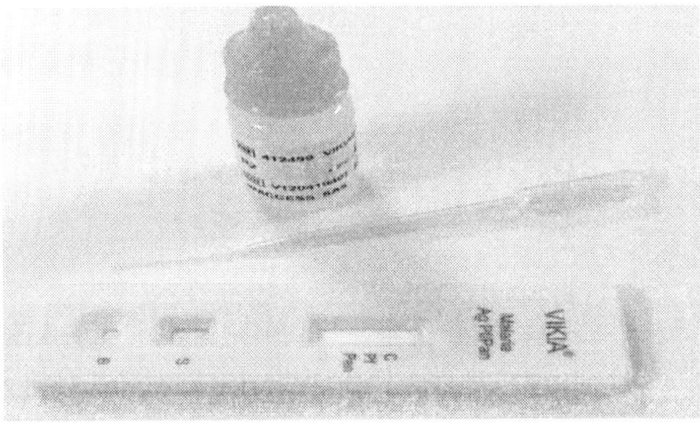

Figure 8. Design of VIKIA Malaria Ag Pf/PanTM test. (Adopted from Menard et al.)

It is easy to use, interpret and simple to store, not requiring a cold chain system.

SD Malaria Antigen Malaria Pf 05FK90-02-0 (HRP2/PLDH)

This RDT was developed by Standard Diagnostic Inc. Korea and is made of 3-bands constituting a control line, a test line with antibodies directed to PfHRP2 and a different test line with antibody directed to Pf-pLDH. In a study, Huemeker et al. found that it performed very well for P *falciparum* diagnosis. The combination of PfHRP2 and Pf-pLDH ensures a low detection threshold and counters the potential problems of PfHRP2 detection such as gene deletion and prozone effect.

Chapter V

Update in Malaria Treatment and Resistance

Pharmacological Properties of Antimalarial Drugs

The pharmacological basis of antimalarial drugs is for therapeutic use. This ranges from their mechanism of action to pharmacokinetics. These properties are briefly described below.

Mechanisms of Action

i) Folate pathway: Agents like Sulphadoxine/pyrimethamine (SP) and Chlorproguanil-dapsone (Lapdap) are competitive inhibitors of the folate pathway. The main problem with these agents is that point mutation easily develops making resistance to antifolate drugs very rapid.

ii) Mitochondria function: Atovaquone inhibits the cytochrome c reductase. Just like the antifolate group of drugs, resistance rapidly develops within the mitochondria; there are potential targets such as dihydroorotate dihydrogenase.

iii) Hemoglobin digestion in food vacuole: 4-aminoquinolines interferes with the hemoglobin digestion process. Other food vacuole processes such as plamepsin aspartic proteinases and falcipain cysteine proteinase are also possible drug targets.

iv) Alkylating agents: Artemisinin drugs generate free radicals that alkylate the membrane of the parasite. It has been postulated that this process maybe catalyzed by haemozoin. Earlier it was suggested that the parasite finds it difficult to develop a resistance but resistant cases have been reported in some areas.

v) Apicoplast: Certain antibiotics such as tetracyclines interfere with protein translation by working in the apicoplast.

Overview of Main Drug Classes

The main groups of antimalarial drugs are briefly described below.

- Chloroquine was the first-line of drugs used throughout Africa until resistance to it forced the WHO to recommend its replacement. Chloroquine resistance is associated with the reduced accumulation of the drug. The intra-erythrocytic malaria survives by consuming hemoglobin, detoxifying heme by polymerization to haemozoin or malaria pigment. This process is inhibited by the drug and other related arylamino alcohols.
- Amodiaquine is a close relative of chloroquine. As a result, cross-resistance between the two has been reported. Studies have shown that a larger proportion of patients given amodiaquine experience a cure than when chloroquine is used. Amodiaquine has been found to have an advantage over artemisinin drugs when in combination.
- Antifolate drugs are always used in fixed-ration combination and the most common is Sulphadoxine/pyrimethamine (SP). This group acts by interfering with DNA synthesis through depletion of the pool of tetrahydrofolate, an important co-factor. Three fundamental points needs to be highlighted: 1. One structurally diverse group of molecules acts as competitive inhibitors of dihydrofolate reductase (DHFR) which is an enzyme. The group includes pyrimethamine and biguanides proguanil and chlorcycloguanil for their action on DHFR; 2. Another group of molecules acts as competitive inhibitors of the dihydropteroate (DHPS), an earlier enzyme of folate pathways and which has been found lacking in mammals. The group includes sulphonamides, principally

sulphadoxine and sulphalene as well as sulphone which is exclusively dapsone and 3. The DHFR inhibitors have some therapeutic utility if used alone as found in cases involving proguanil chemoprophylaxis but not the case for DHPS inhibitors. For malaria treatment, DHFR inhibitors and DHPS inhibitors are used in synergistic combination. Series of fixed combinations such as SP and pyrimethamine/dapsone have been available for sometime while chlorproguanil /dapsone was introduced towards the end of 2003. SP was also used across Africa for the treatment of chloroquine –resistant *falciparum* malaria but resistance rapidly developed and a severe skin reaction led to its discontinuation for chemoprophylaxis. SP has a long elimination half-life which can be the basis for selective pressure for resistance as new infections are exposed to eventual sub-inhibitory drug concentrations. Pyrimethamine is well absorbed after oral or intramuscular administration. The elimination half-life in children with malaria is between 81 and 124 hours after oral and intramuscular administration respectively. Proguanil and chlorproguanil which can only be given orally can reach their peak concentration in plasma after 2 to 4 hours. Dapsone when combined with pyrimethamine is occasionally used for prophylaxis but the development of agranulocytosis has limited its use. Proguanil can be formulated alone for chemoprophylaxis and also in fixed-ration combination with atovaquone. It has little value in malaria endemic areas due to its high cost. Some adverse events have been associated with this group of drugs. Severe allergic reactions to sulphur drugs is well documented. In slowly eliminated drugs such as sulphadoxine, this can be life threatening. Dapsone is associated with a range of concentration-dependant and idiosyncratic adverse reactions. Patients with severe G6PD deficiency may develop severe hemolysis and methemoglibinaemia. Allergies to dapsone clinically manifest as rash and fever. Finally, patients given pyrimethaminc-dapsonc twice weekly as prophylaxis for malaria develop bone marrow reactions. Pyrimethamine and the biguanides proguanil as well as chlorproguanil are said to be associated with little skin toxicity.

- Quinine
- Mefloquine is an expensive drug which acts against the asexual stage of all the species of the human malaria parasite. It has some problems such as causing nausea and vomiting. It is also eliminated slowly with a half-life ranging between 15 to 33 days. A steady state is reached after 8 weeks of weekly dosing in prophylaxis settings and this can be the basis

for the development of resistance. Mefloquine is used for prophylaxis and treatment of uncomplicated multi-drug resistant falciparum malaria. When it is co -administered with artesunate, it has proven effect against uncomplicated falciparum malaria in areas that have a high-level resistance to mefloquine alone. Dose related adverse events, normally mild, are common and in most cases involves the gastrointestinal (GIT). Serious central nervous system (CNS) events such as headaches, dizziness, insomnia and depression have been reported and vary between 1.8 to 7.6%. It is normally higher in females than males. When used in pregnancies, it increases the risk of stillbirths. The British BNF advises the exclusion of pregnancy before the commencement of mefloquine treatment.

- Atovaquone has a unique mode of action as it inhibits the transportation of the cytochrome electron. Atovaquone is normally not used alone in the treatment of malaria infection but in fixed combination with proguanil. The two have been found to be synergistic. Proguanil does not act in this combination as a pro-drug for the DHFR inhibitor cycloguanil. It is rather the parent compound that synergizes through a yet to be defined mechanism of action. This is important as 3-5% of Africans and Caucasians as well as 13-23% of Asians cannot convert proguanil to cycloguanil as they posses polymorphism in the gene encoding cytochrome P450 2C19. Atovaquone/proguanil is highly effective in all populations but yet also expensive.
- Halofantrine is sometimes used for uncomplicated but multi-drug resistant falciparum malaria. Its absorption is incomplete and varies; for example its bioavailability increases after the ingestion of fatty food. The drug is eliminated with a terminal half-life of 1 to 2 days. Its most adverse effect is the prolongation of ECG OT intervals and the resulting ventricular arrhythmias.
- Artemisinin is a potent antimalaria compound derived from the plant *Artemesia annua.* The artemisinin compounds act by haem-catalyzed intraparasitic production of highly reactive carbon-centered free radicals due to the breakdown of the peroxide bridge within the sesquiterpene lactone molecule. Hemazoin is thought to catalyze the decomposition of these drugs which may explain the large therapeutic index seen in these drugs. Unlike other antimalarial agents, the artemisinins have marked effects on the circulating forms of the parasite. They generally have gametocytocidal effects on *P. falciparum.* Certain hemoglobinopathies

have been found to be associated with a reduction in the antimalarial activities of artemisinin. This is because of the reduced intra-erythocytic availability of iron to catalyze the opening of peroxide bridge.

What Is Available Now?

The drugs now used in malaria therapy are Artemisinin-based combination therapy (ACT) which is now the main backbone of malaria treatment. It is responsible for a global reduction of malaria infection. It is extracted from plant material and various semi synthetic derivatives such as Artemether, artesunate and dihydroartemisinin presently in clinical use. They are used in the treatment of severe malaria although they are usually combined with other drugs for the treatment of uncomplicated falciparum malaria. The group is well tolerated and potent. Some resistance cases have been reported.

Mode of Action

The mechanism of action is not fully understood but there has been some postulation. It has been suggested that the breakdown of the labile peroxide bridge within the sesquiterpene lactone molecule leads to the generation of free radicals that alkylates the parasite membrane rapidly while hemozoin is suggested to catalyze the decomposition of these drugs. It is believed that this might be the reason why this drug group has a large therapeutic index. It has been found that *P berghei* which do not possess hemozoin are resistant to artemisinins. Because of their short-life, they are not useful in prophylaxis. They do not have any effect on the hepatic stage of neither the parasite, nor relapsing malaria. The artemisinins have gametocytocidal effects on *P falciparum* and are useful in treating CM associated with *falciparum* malaria. The recurrence rate is over 40% when treatment is for 1-3 days but considerably less when treatment is extended over 7 days.

Clinical Pharmacokinetics

Artemisinin and its derivatives can be administered by several routes. The water soluble derivative artesunate can be given by the oral, intramuscular (IM), intravenous (IV) and even intrarectal routes. They are rapidly hydrolyzed in vivo to dihydroartemisinin (DHA). It has also been found that it is rapidly absorbed and extensively metabolized in vitro by the cytochrome P450 (CYP) enzymes into DHA. All members of the group have a short elimination time. Arthemether absorption has been found to be slower with lower biotransformation to DHA when administered by either IM or IV routes than when given by the anal route. Pregnancy has been reported to alter the pharmacokinetics of this group and other antimalarial drugs. Artesunates have a short elimination half time (<10 minutes). The metabolites are important in exerting antimalaria effects because the elimination half-time is somehow longer (approximately 1 hour). The relatively short half-time for elimination of DHA has the advantage that drug-resistant selection is less likely. However, it has been predicted that it can potentially be associated with the risk of recrudescence when these drugs are used as monotherapy. Oral artesunate is rapidly absorbed in an uncomplicated manner with good bioavailability.

Formulation of ACT Available

For the first-line treatment of uncomplicated *P falciparum* malaria worldwide, the WHO recommends the use of Artemisinin (ART) Combined Therapy (ACT). In defining the properties of these ART derivatives, factors such as their ability to rapidly decrease the number of asexual blood stage parasites, their activity against the broadest range of intraerythrocytic development stages and their ability to inhibit the development of mature sexual stage parasites are taken into consideration. Different formulations of ACT have been developed. Most of these formulations are fixed-dosed co-formulations (Table 6) which facilitate adherence, convenience and misuse prevention. These combinations, in most cases, provide a cure with a 3 day treatment regimen and also protect against the emergence of resistance to the ART derivatives. ART have shown an excellent safety profile in humans. Various studies have been undertaken to compare the efficacy and tolerability of these formulations. In a randomized open label study comparing the 2 day-regimen of artequick to a 3-day regimen of coarsucam in both adults and children involving 128 patients concluded that both forms of ACT are highly efficacious in the treatment of uncomplicated *falciparum* malaria. However, although the 2-day course of artequick was equally effective as the 3-day course, the clearance of the parasite and fever were shorter with coarsucam. In another study using dihydroartemisinin-piperaquine and artesunate plus mefloquine in the treatment of uncomplicated *P falciparum* malaria in India, Gargano *et al.* found that parasite and fever clearance was rapid in both treatment groups as summarized in Table 4. They also found that both regimens were well tolerated with most of the adverse events attributed to the malaria episode itself. In Ethiopia, Arthemether-Lumefantrine was introduced in 2004 as the first-line treatment for uncomplicated *falciparum* malaria. ART monotherapy is only curative when administered for 7 days and recrudescence has been found to be common.

Table 6. Drug combinations in use

Artesunate + amodiaquine
Artesunate + sulphadoxine-pyrimethamine
Artemether-lumefantrine
Chloroquine + sulphadoxine-pyrimethamine
Amodiaquine + sulphadoxine-pyrimethamine
Artesunate + mefloquine
Chlorprogaunil - dapsone
Artesunate-pyronaridine
Dihydroartemisinine-piperaquine (Artekin®, Duo-Cotecxin®, Euratesim)

Eshetu et al. in an open-labeled study tried to evaluate the effectiveness of AL in the Jimma zone (Ethiopia). Their study which involved 348 patients showed that AL was well tolerated and effective in the Jimma zone of Ethiopia. However, the recrudescence rate at day 42 for children under the age of 5 years was 9.4%. This means regular monitoring should be implemented in conformity to the recommendation by the WHO. These studies and others have shown that ACT is effective and well tolerated. In most of the cases there were some serious adverse events which were attributed to the malaria episode itself but these need further assessment. Outside of Africa where *P vivax* is the most common cause of human malaria infections, Arthermether-lumefantrine has been found to be a good treatment option when combined with primaquine.

Is ACT safe in pregnant women? This question is essential as any doubt in the use of ACT may result in the public losing confidence in a drug leading to a lack of adherence. This will then ultimately result in treatment failure and the development of drug resistance. Current guidelines allowing the inclusion of pregnant women in clinical studies varies from the U.S. Food& Drug Administration's (FDA) cautious attitude to the Joint United Nations Programme on HIV/AIDS (UNAIDS) advocating for the inclusion of pregnant women. The data available are mostly non-clinical versions. Animal studies have shown some adverse effects of Artemisinin derivatives. Some studies have been undertaken to fill the 'clinical data' gap. In a pharmacovigilance study by Rulisa et al., they found that when pregnant women in their second and third trimester periods are exposed to artemether-lumefantrine, there was no specific concern in relation to the treatment regimen. However, there were some complications which they attributed to the malaria episode itself. Further studies in all stages of pregnancy are required to really draw the line on the safety profile of using ACT during pregnancy.

ACT has generally been found to be safe despite several reports on the neurotoxic effects of artheether and artemether. Neurotoxicity has been seen in animals but has yet to be seen in humans after a high dose of these compounds. A longer recovery time from coma in CM patients has been observed in those treated with IM artemether compound when compared to IM quinine.

Despite the huge success in the reduction of malaria infection, there have been documented cases of treatment failure with ACT. Farnet et al. reported of AL-treatment failure in a traveler with *P falciparum* malaria after returning from Tanzania. Similar treatment failures were reported from travelers who went to Sierra Leone and Congo. In the report of Farnet et al., mefloquine was used to resolve the AL-treatment failure. A similar outcome was reported by Rolling et al. Several studies have provided evidence of cases of emerging artemisinin resistance along the Thai-Mayamar border while the situation remains critical along the Thai-Cambodian border.

When can treatment be referred to as a failure? The WHO in its 2003 guidelines defined treatment outcomes as follows: Early treatment failure is the development of severe malaria on days 1, 2, or 3 in the presence of parasitaemia, day-2 parasitaemia higher than day 0, day-3 parasitaemia greater or equal to 25% of the day 0 count, or the presence of parasitaemia on day 3 and with an auxiliary temperature greater or equal to 37.5°C. Late treatment failure is the development of severe malaria after day 3, the presence of parasitaemia and fever after day 3, or the presence of parasitaemia after day 7 irrespective of temperature. Adequate clinical and parasitological response (ACPR) is the absence of parasitaemia on day 28 and not meeting the criteria for early or late treatment failure. The issue of drug resistance will be dealt with later.

Limitation of Artemisinins

Aside from the issue of costs, there are some problems with the current artemisinins as outlined below:

1) Used as a monotherapy, it has poor cure rate
2) It has a neurotoxic effect
3) It is also associated with transient gastrointestinal tract disturbance and some rare cases of allergic reactions or hemolysis. An important concern is fetotoxicity based on animal studies. However, it has not shown to be teratogenic in the small amount of human data that is available.

Mechanism of Drug Resistance

The WHO defines drug resistance as "the ability of the parasite strain to survive or multiply in the presence of drug concentrations that normally destroy parasites of the same species or prevent their multiplication, provided that the drug was properly absorbed and the parasites exposed to it". Antimalarial drug resistance is usually due to spontaneous development of mutants selected by antimalarial drugs concentration that result in the development of differential mutants to distinct genetic parasite types. Drug resistance in malaria infection is either due to changes in drug accumulation or efflux as seen in chloroquine, amodiaquine, quinine, mefloquine and halofantrine resistance or reduction in affinity for the drug target as a result of point mutation in the gene encoding for the target; for example pyrimethamine and atovoquone resistance. In bacteria, other mechanisms of drug resistance have been identified such as transferable resistance genes, drug destroying enzymes and the activation of accessory pathways. However, they do not appear in antimalarial drugs resistance.

Chloroquine resistance has been found to be a result of reduced parasite accumulation of the drug. Resistance to CQ is due to a reduction of drug concentration in the parasite's food vacuole. It is hypothesized that CQ resistance involves a multigenic process in which natural resistance is associated with polymorphism in the 36 Kb segment of the parasite's chromosome 7 which contains *cg2*, a polymorphic gene encoding a 330kDa protein. Several molecular markers of *P falciparum* resistance have been identified. A K76T allele has been described in the CQ resistance transporter gene (*pfcrt*) and is associated with treatment failure in CQ and amodiaquine therapies; 486 alleles of multidrug resistance gene 1 (*pfmdr1*) have also been described, and associated with CQ and amodiaquine resistance. Dihydrofolate reductase (*dhfr*) and dihydropteroate synthase (*dhps*) mutation has been linked with resistance in SP drugs. Mutation associated with antifolate resistance has been described in codons 436,437,540,581 and 613 in the *pfdhps* gene and codon 108, 51, 59, 140, 16 and 164 in the *pfdhfr* gene. A quintuple mutation of *pfdhr* (S108N, N511 and C59R1 and *pfdhps* (A437G and K540E) have been described and linked with the risk of treatment failure. These have been suggested to be the molecular markers of SP treatment failure in patients with uncomplicated *P falciparum*.

In Sub-Saharan Africa, *dhfr* mutant (Asn-108/IIe-51/Arg-59) has been described. *Dhps* double mutation (Gly-439/Gly-540) is now strongly associated with resistance to antifolate while Leu-164 mutation is a major contributor to the rapid spread of antifolate resistance in Africa. The dhps mutation at Condon 581 is associated with therapeutic failure and a *dhps* triple mutant allele (A437G/K540E/AS81G) has been confirmed in Tanzania and is increasing in prevalence. A recent study identified mutation at *dhfr* 164, dhps. In artemisinin treatment failure, the sarcol endoplasmic reticulum Ca^{2+} ATPase (*pfatp6*) might have a role. Specific point mutation in codons 769, 623 and 431 is associated with artemisinin resistance.

Table 7. Types of haplotypes of SNPs in P falciparum isolates in Yunnan Province China (Source: Huang et al.)

Gene	Haplotype
Pfdhfr	151 R59 N108 L164
Pfdhps	151/R59/N108 A436 G437 E540 G581 G437/E540
Pfdhfr/pfdhps	151/R59/N108+ G437/E540

Mefloquine resistance in most cases is associated with mutation in or amplification of ATP-dependent P-glycoprotein pump homologue which is encoded by the MDR gene family. It has been found that resistance to mefloquine develops rapidly when compared to chloroquine. In a study by Nosten et al. in Thailand, they found that there was a significant emergence of resistance within 6 years after mefloquine was first introduced. Table 7 highlights some of the existing mutations in Yunnan province associated with *P falciparum* infection.

In vivo artemisinin resistance has been proposed and identified as a result of a significant decrease of the parasite reduction rate which manifested clinically marked by longer parasite clearance from the body. One such proposal is the interaction with sarcoplasmic Ca^{2+} ATPase 6. In naturally occurring polymorphism in pfatp6 in the field isolate, it has been suggested that polymorphism at codon 769 might be associated with a reduction in susceptibility of these isolates to artemether.

In *P vivax* infection, a single nucleotide polymorphism at codon Y976f *(pvmdr1)* has been described in *P vivax* resistance to chloroquine. Available data suggests that point mutation at codon Y976F and F1076L of *pvmdr1* is associated with resistance to 4-aminoquinolones, chloroquine and amodiaquine. No association of mutant F1076L with chloroquine has yet to be reported but common *pvmdr1* haplotypes found in nature are F1076L and Y976F plus F1076L while the single mutant Y976F has rarely been reported. As a result of this data, it is believed that there is a 2-step mutational path with mutation at F1076LL followed by Y976F leading to chloroquine resistance although in vivo substitution of the theory is required. It has also been argued that polymorphism in the copy number of the pvmdr1 gene can also result in drug resistance in *P vivax*. This is supported by a link between gene amplification and decreased in vitro susceptibility to mefloquine, artesunate and amodiaquine but increased susceptibility to chloroquine. In regards to the use of SP in *P vivax* infection, SP has not been indicated for treatment of *vivax* infection but evidence supports the argument that intensive SP treatment in *falciparum* infection may also select resistant *P vivax* in regions where both coexist. Due to the importance of *P vivax* infection, molecular markers should be used in monitoring the effects of SP pressure on the parasite. It has also been suggested that mutation in codon I13L, P33L, F57L/I, S58R, T61M, S117N/T and I173L/F might confer resistance to pyrimethamine in *P vivax*. In addition, in vitro analysis of *pvdhfr* revealed some mutation which confers resistance to antifolate, resulting in reduction in drug affinity to the target enzyme. *P vivax dhps* mutation at codon S382A/C, A383G, K523M/T/C and A53G/A are believed to result in resistances to sulphadoxine. Others have reported primaquine treatment failure in *P vivax*. Although the authors attributed it to polymorphism in the human cytochrome P-450 isoenzyme

2D6 (CYD2D6) which resulted in reduced metabolism of primaquine, more studies need to be conducted to understand the molecular mechanism of resistance in *vivax* infection.

Techniques in Identifying Resistance

Measuring antimalarial drug resistance is very important. Antimalarial drug resistance and drug efficacy can be monitored by performing therapeutic studies, measurement of drug concentration in the blood, in-vitro analysis that monitors the parasite's phenotypic changes as well as analyzing the molecular markers associated with genetic changes. Due to recent advances in molecular techniques, analysis and monitoring of genetic markers is now an alternative for the detection of drug resistance. Studies have shown that identification of SNPs and gene duplication which has been associated with antimalarial drug resistance has been utilized in the evaluation of resistance to treatment. The techniques used in detecting SNPs are primarily PCR based. After the amplicons have been obtained, the presence of SNPs can be detected by restriction fragment length polymorphism (RFLP), DNA sequencing or single stranded conformation polymorphism. Other methods can also be used, such as a single nucleotide primer extension (SNPE), melting curve analysis in fluorescence resonance energy transfer (FRET-MCA), molecular beacon, melting probe hybridization, real-time PCR and microarray. Each of these methods has been found to have some advantages and disadvantages. However, there is still the need to develop new SNPs analysis techniques which improve the existing techniques. Some of the desirable qualities for the next generation of SNPs analysis techniques include improved accuracy and sensitivity, fast turnover, reduced price as well as high throughput capability. Applied Biosystem has recently introduced TaqMan Allelic Discrimination assays which detect SNPs associated with antimalarial drug resistance. Data has shown that this assay is capable of detecting mixed alleles. However, it must be noted that this PCR based assay discriminates the presence of either allele based on affinity of one probe to the SNP sequence of the allele present as opposed to the one absent. Therefore, some SNP assays might detect mixed infection better than others which depend on the chemistry of each probe.

Another approach for sensitivity assay is non-radioisotope histidine-rich protein-2 (HRP-2) ELISA, a relatively sensitive assay which can measure 50% inhibitory concentration (IC50) values for *P falciparum* isolates and can be used for detecting drug resistance in malaria infection. This assay has been found to be safer, more expedient and less costly than other radioisotope assays. The HRP-2 ELISA assay was developed by the Armed Forces Research Institute of Medical Sciences (AFRIMS) with the aim of providing a simple, objective, easily reproducible test system which includes the advantages of the currently available techniques while excluding most of their disadvantages. Since 2004, AFRIMS has routinely applied this assay for 'immediate ex vivo' (IEV) during susceptibility testing using a fresh field isolate without culture adaptation from multidrug resistant areas in Cambodia and Thailand. AFRIMS selected the "Indochina" W2 clone as the reference for its genetic similarity to potential field isolates, its drug susceptibility profile and ease of cultural adaptation. This assay has been found to generate IC50 results which are comparable to the World Health Organization's (WHO) microplate schizont maturation test and [^{3}H]-hypoxanthine uptake. In comparison with the schizont maturation test, the HRP-2 has the advantage of being rapid and also does not involve the use of any radioisotopes. In addition, measuring drug sensitivity on fresh isolates with culture adaptation provides accurate results. They mirror an overall drug susceptibility phenotype of in vivo infection and avoid the loss of drug resistant parasite subpopulation drug culture adaptation. The HRP-2 assay can be utilized for a wide variety of applications, ranging from epidemiology to the screening of new drugs and the potential to replace the traditional in vitro techniques. The complete HRP-2 assay takes 2.5 hours to perform, may be carried out with commercial test kits and requires less technical equipment. However, a global HRP-2 reference assay needs to be developed. HRP-2 has a long half –life in vivo, therefore coupled with its persistence in patients who have been successfully treated with falciparum malaria limits its application on HRP-2 based rapid text for monitoring therapeutic efficacy, although its stability can be regarded as an advantage. The amount of HRP-2 found in culture samples has been found to be associated with parasite growth which increases with parasite development and multiplication. Noedl et al. therefore concluded in a study that HRP-2 might be used as an excellent marker for parasite growth and its inhibition by antimalarial drugs.

Management of Drug Resistance

The continued expansion of *Plasmodium* resistance to various antimalarial agents is an urgent public health concern. Over the last decade, there has been dramatic progress in the global malaria control and elimination effort. This can be attributed in large part to the scaling-up of vector control interventions and improved access to effective antimalarial therapy especially the use of ACT regimen. Malaria cases have therefore fallen by more than 50% in 43 countries since 2001. Since 2000, the malaria associated mortality rate decreased by more than 25% globally while in Africa, there was a greater than 33% decline. Worldwide, malaria patients depend on ACTS. In 2010, about 180 million ACT courses were procured for the public sector. All of these achievements have been threatened by drug resistance. Managing drug resistance is therefore an important part of the malaria control effort. Many management strategies have been proposed. The identification of factors which result in the emergence of resistance is highly significant.

In Western Cambodia, these factors include 30 years of ART monotherapy which has now been officially banned, drugs that were substandard and/or used sub optimally and parasite genetic backgrounds that favor the emergence of multi drug resistance. Another factor is the low rate of transmission which results in insufficient immunity to eliminate the parasite that might survive drug treatment thereby increasing selective pressure. Others have touted community Direct Observation Therapy (DOT) and follow up as vital in reducing the spread of potential multi-drug resistance. Identification of the early warning signs of drug resistance and treatment by DOT for first-line and second-line village malaria workers (VMWs) is a feasible approach. Say et al. proposed that to ensure high quality results, strong monitoring, supervision and real-time feed-back results are needed in this direction. Therefore, they suggested that further discussion is needed to: 1. Develop a comprehensive strategy to expand surveillance on a large scale including improving malaria case management and follow-up; 2. Develop harmonized guidelines for promoting cross-border treatment and contact tracing and 3. Simplify the strategy for second-line treatment and screening surrounding an index case.

Another management strategy is containment of the malaria parasite developing resistance to antimalarial drugs. The WHO suggested the Global Plan for Artemisinin Resistance Containment in 2010 with the aim of containing or better eliminating resistance parasites in the Greater Mekong sub-region. The expected outcome of this effort will prevent the further spread of artemisinin-resistant parasites to other regions. Routine monitoring must also be strengthened to enable early detection of resistance in malaria therapy especially artemisinin resistance to ensure that first 0 line ACT are effective and can allow for timely change in treatment policies. Most importantly, a dynamic open access database needs to be established which would include molecular markers and patterns of antimalarial drug resistance.

Stages of Drug Development

Below is a brief description of the various stages in drug development.

Preclinical Studies

This is the initial phase of drug development where the toxicology parameters of the drug are analyzed in animals. The activities of this phase include: 1. Studies of the drug's mode of action and detailed pharmacological profile, 2. Toxicology studies (single-dose); 3. Additional toxicology studies (repeated-dose); 4. Reproduction studies involving both sexes and fertility studies examining any embryotoxicity and teratogenicity effects and 5. Mutagenesis studies.

Phase 1 Human Studies

All phases of human studies must conform to good clinical practice regulations. This phase may be carried out on healthy adults normally comprising either sexes or a patient with the diseases. The total number of participants is 100 and the main aims are 1. Investigate the safety profile and 2. Pharmacokinetics studies where a comparison is made of the human data with what was observed with the animals.

Phase II Human Studies

Here an open-label assessment of the new drug in patients is made. During this phase, detailed studies are performed with the disease being treated. One of the main elements of this phase is a description of the relationship between the dosage and its effect. There is also some element of pharmacokinetic studies. Drug safety and tolerability is an important feature here. In addition, interactions between the new drug and those which may be co- administered are analyzed. Multiples of 100 patients are used in this phase.

Phase III Human Studies

These involve large, randomized clinical studies to evaluate the efficacy, safety and tolerability of the new drug that is compared with those on either placebo or standard medication. The number of patients in this phase ranges from 1,000 to 2,000. Therefore in most cases, the adverse event profile of the new drug is unknown when launched. Compliance with the administration of the drug is closely monitored during this phase.

Phase IV Human Studies

Once the quality standard has been met and the studies have proven that the new drug is efficacious and tolerable as well the safety profile having been ascertained after rigorous studies involving up to 2,000 patients, the national authorities do not have enough information to make a decision of splicing the new drug (in this sense the antimalarial drug) into policy. The main areas needed when assessing the operational use of a new drug especially in Africa are safety, compliance, effectiveness and drug resistance.

New Drugs and Novel Strategies in the Pipeline

There has been a tremendous transformation in the landscape of malaria drug discovery and development. However, in the face of the threat posed by antimalarial drug resistance, there is an urgent need for a new research direction with the identification of a new drug target as the goal. There is a need for new drugs that prevent transmission, stop relapse and provide chemoprotection against new infection. The Target Products Profiles (TPPs) explain the ideal medicine and minimum acceptable profile in malaria therapy. Starting with children under the age of five years, it has been recommended that child-friendly pediatric formulation should be the main priority since 85% of malaria cases occur among that age group. Coartem® Dispersible which was developed in collaboration between Malaria Medicine Venture (MMV) and Novartis is a taste-marked dispersible ACT. Two other pediatric formulations are now in development, which are expected to be submitted in 2013: granule formulation of pyronaridine-artesunate and a dispersible formulation of DHA-piperaquine. Prospective drugs that would target severe malaria are in the pipeline. Most are to be used as adjunct therapy, to be given with schizonticide to reduce the risk of sequelae of severe malaria such as neurologic damage. However, adjunct therapy has generally been shown to be of little benefit. Series of reports on molecules such as N-acetyl cysteine and pentoxifylline failed to show any benefit. An interesting adjunct therapy which just completed Phase I trials is sevuparin (tagged DF-02), a heparin derivative with no anti-coagulation activity that blocks resetting, a very important process in severe malaria. Eisai is also developing a drug for severe malaria in the form of TLR-9 antagonist (E6446).

The new schizonticide being proposed for severe malaria is albitiazolium bromide (SAR97276) which is a choline antagonist. It has poor oral bioavailability. It has been shown in Phase II trials that higher doses are needed for uncomplicated malaria. Formulations using artemisinin derivatives are being developed. Kunming and Sanofi are developing an IM arthemether in conformity with the WHO's guidelines for treating severe malaria. There has been a question regarding the neurotoxicity potential of this drug as seen in preclinical trials involving animals; although this has not been reported in humans. A sublingual spray of arthemether is being produced by Eastland Medical System Ltd/ Proto Pharma which is likely to be used as monotherapy. The WHO special program for research and training in Tropical Diseases is collaborating with UNICEF, UNDP and the World Bank to develop artesunate suppositories as a pre-referral treatment option for severe malaria cases. Clinical studies which involve 12,068 patients showed that this formulation increased the chance of survival of patients more than 6 hours away from hospitals and among the youngest patients when given a 100mg dose.

The demand for artemisinin is very great. It is estimated that to treat all malaria cases, an excess of 200 tons of artemisinin is required every year. This is creating a 'demand' problem for the world as price of the product keeps fluctuating between $300/kg to $1,500/kg. There have also been complaints that the ordering of artemisinin could take up to 2 years before is delivered. There is the need to identify new targets for malaria treatment and find solutions in relation to artemisinin demands. The following three solutions have been proposed: a) use of higher-yielding seeds, b) using yeast for scalable products in bioreactors and c) production of synthetic endoperoxides. In 2000, MMV in collaboration with the University of Nebraska, the Swiss Institute of Tropical Medicine and Monash University began a project with the objective of developing synthetic endoperoxides. OZ277 was the initial product used but it is now referred to as RBx11160 (arterolane). This product showed some activity in a Phase IIa study in uncomplicated *falciparum* malaria but it was found to be inferior to artemisinin. It showed adequate clinical and parasitic response of 60-70% after 7 days treatment as compared to a 95% response with artesunate. OZ277/Rbx11160 was unstable in infected blood and it has been proposed that this might be due to free ferrous iron. Ranbaxy has completed a Phase III study of this combination (OZ277/Rbx11160) at a dose of 150mg and piperaquine at a dose of 750mg. This has been approved in India. MMV has also identified a clinical candidate OZ439 which has been shown to possess superior pharmacokinetics in that exposure was dose –proportional which was similar in patients and volunteers and the plasma concentration remained around the mean parasiticidal concentration for more than 72 hours after a single dose. This means that it has the potential of being a single-dose cure. Phase IIa studies in uncomplicated *P vivax* and *P falciparum* have been completed.

Other synthetic endoperoxides have been developed in the preclinical stage. RKA 182, a tetraoxane has been produced by the University of Liverpool and Liverpool Institute of Tropical Medicine. Preclinical testing showed that it is superior to OZ277. The Central Drug Research Institute in India has also developed CDRI 99/411 which was taken to Phase I study by IPCA but the project has been placed on hold. A trioxane which was fused with 4-aminoquinoline was produced by Palumed while a semi-synthetic endoperoxide artemisone showed good activity in Phase II studies in 2009.

The following products are in line for development:

- Next generation aminoquinolines: A number of 4-aminoquinolines or amino-alcohols are in clinical development. They have been touted as the next generation molecules after ACTs. Phase II studies have been completed on ferroquine in combination with artesunate. In the studies, a total dose as low as 300mg showed clinical activity. Naphtoquine at 400mg when combined with artemisinin also showed some promise. CQ analogs have been synthesized as mono- and bisquinoline-based derivatives and referred to as MAQ and BAQ respectively. Both possess conserved 4-aminoquinoline moiety. A study by Aguiar et al. showed that MAQ and BAQ are active in vitro against CQ-resistant and CQ-sensitive P falciparum at a nanomolar dose.
- New Molecular targets: The prospective of exploring molecular targets in malaria therapy resulted in two compounds being tried in clinical development. The enzyme dihydroorotate dehydrogenase (DHODH) which is known to play an essential role in the survival of the parasite was one of the targets. An inhibitor DSM1 was identified through high throughput screening at the University of Texas, USA. Recently, a new improved version of the inhibitor DSM265 entered the preclinical development phase. In addition, a new generation of dihydrofolate reductase inhibitors has entered the preclinical development. There is one fear associated with this potential inhibitor: how do we deal with potential preexisting mutations in dihydrofolate reductase as a result of wide spread use of pyrimethamine? Work is ongoing to take care of this fear. An inhibitor of purine nucleoside phosphorylase, BCX4945 which was meant for other indications is being promoted for use in malaria therapy although it has not shown any activity in mouse models. It has

also been reported that inhibiting calpain, a calcium-regulate enzyme can be of antimalarial benefit. In addition, fibrates such as gemfibrozil and fenofibrates which are agonists of peroxisome proliferation-activated receptor alpha (PPARα) are used in clinical settings as potent lipid-modifying drugs have been tried for use as an antimalaria agent. A study using fibrates in malaria showed that clofibrate directly inhibited the development of parasitemia in *P berghei*-infected mice. A study by Wong et al. using the following fibrates: fenofibrate, clofibrate, gemfibrozil and fenofibric acid showed that all the fibrates had antimalaria activity with fenobric acid being the most potent. However, the study showed the four fibrates had weak activity in comparison to conventional antimalaria drugs in vitro. It was therefore suggested that fenobric acid could be used in conjunction with other compounds such as DHA. A recent study by Hanson et al. found that Torins when developed as a ATP competitive mammalian target of rapamycin (mTOR) kinase inhibitors has a fast acting antiplasmodial properties that unexpectedly directly target the parasite and block the dynamic trafficking of the proteins of the parasite exported protein 1 (EXP1) and upregulated in sporozoites 4 (UIS4) to the liver stage parasitophorous vacuole membrane (PVM). This leads to the efficient elimination of the parasite by the hepatocytes. They proposed that due to the fact that torin mediated inhibition of the parasite in the liver stage indicates that the compound has a distinct mode of action when compared with the current antimalarial agents in use. This study is essential since it paves the way for the scientific community to develop a new strategy for antimalaria agents especially in this era of resistance. This is because the PVM is an important joint between the malaria parasite and the host cell environment

- New Compounds from cellular screening: There has been advocacy for the direct screening of the whole parasite. This has resulted in the screening of about six million compounds against the intra-erythrocytic phase of the parasite. The result is identification of about 30,000 compounds which showed some activity at the micro molar levels. Spiroindolone NITD609 was developed by Novartis Institute of Tropical Diseases in Singapore in collaboration with the Swiss Tropical and Public Health Institute and the Dutch Biomedical Primate Research Center. It is now in Phase IIa clinical studies. Imidazolopiperazine GNF156 was also identified which showed some in vitro potency against blood, liver schizont and gametocyte stage of the *Plasmodium* but not the hypnozoites. It has an oral efficacy in mouse malaria models and now in human volunteers' studies.

- Natural Products: Interest keeps growing in natural products and their potential as antimalarial agents. This is not new as the three mainstreams used for malaria therapy come from natural products: quinine, lapachol (led to atovaquone) and artemisinin. Extracts of *Bidens pilosa* have been found to be active against the malaria parasite both in vivo and in vitro. Other natural products such as fungi are used as a source of new drugs from which secondary metabolites that have antimalaria activity can be isolated. Pycnidione, isolated from the marine fungus, *Ploma* species have been shown to exhibit significant activity against *P falciparum*. There are many traditionally used plants across Africa and the Amazon regions which have not been screened for antimalaria activity and little is known about their chemical composition. This makes them an interesting avenue for further exploration.
- Use of antibiotic for malaria treatment: for e.g. use of quinolone as antimalaria with dual mechanism of action against two respiratory enzymes NADH: ubiquine oxidoreductase (*P falciparum*) and cytochrome bc. Clindamycin is also recommended with AS for second-line antimalarial treatment. Fosmidomycin, a natural antibacterial agent has been tried in clinical studies. It inhibits 1-deoxy-D-xylulose 5-phosphate reductoisomerase, an enzyme which is involved in the synthesis of isoprenoids and found to be essential for the survival of the parasite. Azithromycin, a macrolide antibiotic has been found to affect the growth of *P falciparum* by targeting the apicoplast 50S ribosomal subunit and inhibits protein synthesis in this organelle. Geldanamycin, a benzoquinone ansamycin also showed antimalarial activity by inhibiting the heat shock protein HSP90, a molecular chaperone that is important for the maturation of proteins that promotes the survival and growth of dividing cells.
- Control of Transmission-blocking Agents: Effective control of malaria requires continuous development of new preventive and management strategies. Most of the effective drugs available now target the asexual stage of the parasite thereby still allowing the transmission of the circulating gametocyte from humans to mosquitoes; with data showing that the potential of malaria transmission remains high even after the administration of agents that target the asexual stage of the parasite when the gametocyte prevalence and density are low. This is a major problem

in malaria control as circulating gametocytes that are infectious to mosquitoes persist weeks after treatment. Primaquine and ACT all have antigametocyte activity but have some defects in regards to preventing malaria transmission in mosquitoes. Primaquine kills mature but not immature gametocytes while ACT kills immature but not mature gametocytes respectively. It has been presented that the longer utilization of primaquine can kill all gametocytes but such a strategy results in GIT intolerance in some individuals and hemolysis in patients with G6PD deficiency. These data support the need for the development of transmission blocking drugs for effective malaria control. Some studies have tried to develop novel transmission-blocking agents. A study by Ojo et al. showed that a new class of transmission-blocking compounds, bumped kinase inhibitors (BKIs) had an inhibitory effect on the microgametocyte exflagellation of *Plasmodium*. Oocysts formation and sporozoite production essential for transmission to mammals were inhibited in mosquitoes which were fed with either BKI-1-treated human blood or mice treated with BKI-1. The mechanism of action of BKI is believed to be inhibiting *Plasmodium* calcium-dependent kinase 4 but have little activity against mammalian kinase. The author's data showed that when used in combination with drugs active against the asexual stage, BKI could be an ideal tool for malaria control. However, one mitigating factor is the emergence of resistance, although it is hypothesized that the emergence of resistance is less than when asexual stages are targeted. More studies need to be done to evaluate the molecular mechanism of action and resistance pattern of BKI. Another novel approach is the utilization of TCA cycle inhibitors as transmission-blocking agents since the TCA cycle has been proven to be essential for the development of gametocytes. Table 8 lists some of the compounds with potential transmission-blocking activities.

Table 8. Some potential agents for transmission-blocking

Compound	Target
NSC-158011	Phosphoethanolamine N-methyltransferase
4(1H)-quinolone	Exflagellation of male gametocytes
Peptido sulfonyl fluorides	Plasmodial proteasome
ELQ-300	Mitochondrial cytochrome bc1 complex
Ketotifen	Oocysts development

Table 9. Profile of some investigational studies as of 2013

Agent	Target	Phase	Sponsor/ Status
MMV390048	Multiple points of malaria parasite life cycle	Preclinical	Drug Discovery & Development Center (H3-D), University of Cape Town, S/Africa
Inhaled (i) Nitric Oxide	Cerebral malaria	2	Epicenter
AQ-13	Resistant P falciparum	1	Tulane University Health Sciences Center
Riamet® vs. Malarone	Uncomplicated malaria	4	Assistance Publique Hopitaux de Paris
OZ439	Pharmacokinetics/ Pharmacodynamic study	2	Medicines for malaria venture
ACT KNOW	Knowlesi Malaria (Efficacy study)	3	Menzies School of Health Sciences
Sevuparin/DF02	Uncomplicated malaria (Safety/Efficacy study)	I/II	Dilaforette AB
Mefloquine/ Artesunate Artemether/ lumefantrine	Uncomplicated malaria (Efficacy study)	3	LSHTM
IPTp-SP IPTp-DP ISTp-DP	Pregnant malaria (Efficacy study)	4	Kenya Medical Research Center
Arekin	Uncomplicated falciparum malaria Vivax malaria	3	University of Oxford
KAE609	Cure rate (Safety/Efficacy)	2	Novartis Pharmaceutical

- Novel Strategies: A series of novel combinations have been tried in clinical studies. A fixed-dose combination of azithromycin and CQ is being tried for IPT in pregnant women. Tafenoquine, an 8-aminoquinolone has been shown to have some activity against the dormant liver form of *P vivax* in vitro and blood stages in acute malaria. Pyramax pediatric, child friendly granule formulation of ACT is in Phase IV trials. ASAQ (Artesunate, Amodiaquine, and Winthrop) and Artesunate injection are all in various stages of clinical studies. A combination of β-Artemeter and Lumefantrine in lipidic formulation has been found to have excellent antimalaria activity in male Swiss mice. Plasmodial enoyl-ACP reductase (pfENR) is a crucial enzyme in the plasmodial type II fatty acid synthesis II (FAS II) pathway can be investigated for liver stage of malaria infection. pfENR inhibitors can be used as prophylactic agents in malaria infections. Emetine dihydrocholoride hydrate is an anti-protozoal agent used in intestinal and tissue amebiasis infection but it has been shown to have an inhibitory effect on multi-resistant K1 strain of *P falciparum*. All these strategies and others require further study to understand its mechanism of action as a standalone or combination antimalaria agent(s).

infection as well as biological factors as a result of widespread resistance of the malaria parasite to the most effective and well-tolerated drugs and selection of vector mosquitoes which became resistant to most of the available insectides. If these factors are added to the apathy of people to change, it makes malaria control a challenging venture. Malaria was eradicated in some areas around the world sometime ago but the parasite is making a spectacular comeback. What control measures should be initiated to ideally control malaria? This section deals with some of the promising measures for control. However, before discussing the control of malaria, a summary of the global burden of malaria is given below.

Economic and Social Burden of Malaria

The global burden of malaria is staggering. From the biomedical point of view, the burden of malaria is a function of many issues and various public health disciplines which are defined differently. The epidemiologists define the burden of malaria from a morbidity and mortality point of view. Disability-adjusted life years (DALYs), which are an aggregate measure of premature mortality, morbidity and disability, can be used in analyzing the cost-effectiveness of any major intervention. The WHO, therefore, calculates the burden of malaria and other diseases based on an assessment of global DALYs. Sub-Saharan Africa shows the greatest effect of the disease as highlighted earlier in this book and accounts for more than 90% of the burden, followed by Southeast Asia with about 9% of the global burden. Malaria deaths are responsible for almost 3% of the world's DALYs (greater than10% in Africa). Despite the advances in our understanding of malaria ecology and the subsequent development of various intervention models, more than 50% of the world's population is still exposed to malaria; indicating about a 10% increase over the past decade. However, the episode of global malaria burden has been difficult to quantify due to the substantial percentage of the population in endemic areas with parasitemia at one time. Children less than 5 years of age may have 4-9 or more febrile episodes in a year. A study estimated that outside Southern Africa, up to 4.9 billion febrile events or treatments for malaria take place in Africa every year. Apart from its impact on children and pregnancy, anemia, hypoglycemia, ARD and CM can be the dominant pathology. Malaria has been shown to have an effect on nutrition. Caulfield et al. in a Meta analysis study of the effect of iron supplementation on malaria morbidity concluded that there was a heightened risk of infection and non significant increase in malaria attacks and spleen enlargement with supplements. However, treatment was associated with a significant increase in hemoglobin and a decrease in severe anemia.

The economists look at the burden from qualification of cost; be it direct or indirect and its effects on productivity, natural growth and development.

In Sub-Saharan Africa, households face a high economic burden from malaria. These burdens comprise three components: preventive expenditures, direct and indirect costs of illness. The malaria preventive expenditure includes household spending in the month, insecticide treatment, mosquito nets, insect spray, mosquito coils and repellents and malaria prophylaxis. The direct cost of malaria disease includes medicines, food, transport and accommodation. Finally, indirect cost of the disease is said to be represented by the value of production lost due to the disease and is equal to the time lost from work multiplied by the wage rate. The calculation of time lost from work is the sum of the number of days lost to the disease by those reporting malaria or fever and the hours any adult spends accompanying a sick person who is seeking treatment. It has been estimated that in Africa, the cost of the malaria burden is $12 billion every year resulting in a negative impact on the economy and development. An African family might spend up to 25% of their income on malaria prevention and control. The economic burden of sickness on individual households can be high and sometimes catastrophic especially in poor households. In a review study involving various other studies that measured the economic costs and consequences of sickness for households focusing on malaria, TB and HIV/AIDS, Russell found that sickness imposes a high and regressive cost burden on patients and their families in poor settings. A study suggested that reducing the burden of malaria in Nigeria would help contribute to the economic well-being of communities while poverty reduction would be an essential input in improving health. It, therefore, concluded that it is important for the National Malaria Program in Nigeria and their partners to identify mechanisms that will ensure that the poorest have access to essential health interventions.

From the sociological point of view, the burden of malaria is the cost to society imposed by the existence of the disease. It has been suggested that malaria causes changes in household behavior which results in broad social costs such as decisions related to reproduction, education and economic matters. This is believed to have a long-term effect on economic growth and development. The sociocultural factors such as social organization, culturally defined social roles and cultural beliefs about the disease, all play a part in the variability associated with the burden of malaria. Jones and Williams argued that culture, beliefs and political dimensions play roles in the perceptions, individual beliefs, social structure and social action. Social burden affects the biomedical burden of malaria. Societal perceptions influence the willingness of people to change their health behavior. In addition, political and economic interventions, social organization and cultural rules affect people's ability to change behavior. A concept of social vulnerability has been developed which shows the importance of social factors that make some groups or individuals more susceptible to infection or more vulnerable to the consequences of infection. For example, women may have some limitations in their access to funds and the ability to make decisions on their own thereby affecting their ability to seek treatment of a sick child. A study, therefore, argued that understanding the sociocultural model of the burden of malaria is important to the development of intervention which is important for accessing vulnerable people.

Can We Eradicate Malaria?

When HIV/AIDS was first identified, the then U.S. Secretary of Health promised the world that an effective vaccine would soon be available. However, as of this point in time (2013) such a vaccine has not been developed. Is it possible to eradicate malaria? Some have referred to the eradication of smallpox as an example of result of a global effort to eradicate infectious diseases just as one scientist once remarked:" We can close the books of infectious diseases". But with smallpox, the eradication success can be attributed to the simplicity of the virus and visible pathologies in patients which allowed for easy monitoring of cases and the application of a useful point of care vaccine. In the past, the eradication strategy through the Global Malaria Eradication Programme (GMEP) resulted in unprecedented control of malaria transmission. However, this ended in 1969. Due to increased funding since 2000, there have been effective intervention activities. The success that has been achieved recently proves that well funded intervention can have immense benefit while the increase of malaria after GMEP underscores one point: any malaria intervention program is fragile and requires sustainable effort. Sustainability is the main factor that would impede any eradication effort. Presently, the world is facing a financial meltdown which has led to many funding agencies either reducing funding for malaria or even canceling it all together. Sub-Saharan Africa which bears the biggest burden of malaria infection is still plagued with economic mismanagement and a high level of corruption. Recently in Ghana, there was a campaign to distribute bed nets but those who were doing the distribution requested money. Those who didn't have it were not given the bed net. In 1972, when malaria was on the rise as a result of the cessation of GMEP, Bruce-Chwatt suggested that one important concept: "resurgence" which he referred to as "the reappearance of new infection in significant numbers after malaria subsided owing to the measures applied to reduce or interrupt transmission". Later Najera et al. clarified this by remarking "A malaria resurgence is actually the return to a state of equilibrium which has been disturbed" by malaria control.

The main threat in malaria eradication is the issue of resurgence. Some factors have been linked to such resurgence. In a study, Cohen et al. found that the single most common suggested cause of malaria resurgence involved a weakening of malaria programs due to the disruption of funding. Others have projected that funding to be used for treatment and prevention efforts would decline over the next several years. Drugs and insecticide resistance are also threats to any global eradication efforts. Apart from the disruption of funding, complacency following successful reduction, disruption by natural disasters or wars as well as improper utilization of technical solutions; for example in Turkey it has been argued that despite resistance, resurgence was linked to "operational deficiencies stemming from administrative and financial constraints". To prevent resurgence, a study in Mauritius provided a recommendation: Intervention should be sustained, have strong leadership, substantial predictable funding, sustained vigilance and a strong prevention of reintroduction (POR) activities.

So what should be the strategy? Elimination strategies should be the key. The WHO defined malaria elimination as a situation where there is zero local transmission while eradication is defined as the permanent zero worldwide incidence of malaria infection. Many factors impede the eradication concept of malaria. Malaria infection is due to a highly complex interplay between three biological systems which comprise more than 30 species of *Anopheles* mosquitoes and five species of Plasmodia that infects human; each with its complex life cycle, environment, habits and pathogenesis profile. When one adds the current global environmental condition which aids in the transmission of the parasites as well as the factors of travelers' malaria which have resulted in malaria being repeatedly reintroduced in areas where malaria control was positive; it makes it difficult to eradicate malaria. For sustainable malaria elimination, vector control is among the key activities that had a significant impact in the reduction of malaria morbidity and mortality in a number of African countries during the last decade. In vector control, the aim is to reduce the vector capacity to a threshold that is required to maintain the malaria infection rate. So far two interventions have been associated with the success achieved in malaria vector control: the use of long-lasting insecticide-treated nets and the indoor residual spraying of long-lasting insecticides. In general, malaria vector control can be implemented using larval source management using lavicide. Larval source management has been successfully used as a primary mosquito control technique in Canada, several U.S. cities, Singapore, Brazil and throughout Europe. It has been argued that both larval and adult vector density can be controlled using environmental management such as permanent infrastructure changes which can create a temporary unfavorable condition for vector breeding.

However, insecticide resistance poses a problem and has been reported in about 64 countries, mostly in Sub-Saharan Africa and India. A number of countries now depend on the use of DDT as a viable vector control tool. However, the continuous dependence on DDT is environmentally unsustainable due to insecticide resistance as well as the potential health and environmental risks. The use of DDT or its breakdown by-product DDE is associated with some health problems such as menstrual cycle alteration, liver and testicle cancers, breast cancer during pre-pubertal exposure, fetal loss in women in countries that recently used DDT, reduced childhood or pubertal growth after prenatal or early exposure to DDE, DNA damage and apoptosis and neurodevelopment in children up to the age of four. Other health problems which have been postulated to be associated with DDT or DDE usage but with inconclusive evidence include: lung/pancreatic endometrial or prostate cancer, non-Hodgkin's lymphoma, diabetogenic effects, crytorchidims, immunotoxicity, anogentical distance or hypospadias. However, there was no significant association between DDT or DDE and fetal growth development. Preventing mosquito bites and killing the mosquito after they have bitten an individual is another key intervention to be employed in vector control.

No matter the strategy adopted by a community, monitoring which is defined as the systematic tracking of program activities over time and evaluation, defined as the examination of program progress and its determinants; is highly critical. Monitoring and evaluation would require improved system management, improved identification of those infected, improved information sharing for advocacy, enhanced methods of engaging and developing community support as well as improved ways to conduction surveillance activities in the private sector.

Global Warming and Malaria

Global warming is a rise in the average temperature of the earth's atmosphere. There is no doubt that the earth's temperature is rising. The Intergovernmental Panel on Climate Change (IPCC) in 2001 reported that the average global air temperature has risen by 0.6^0 C. This is significant from the public health point of view. Global warming is a gradual process which can have a consequential impact over time. The United Nations Framework Convention on Climate Change (UNFCCC) describes global climatic change as "long term changes in commonly measured meteorological parameters over and above natural variations that are directly or indirectly attributable to human activity resulting in altering the atmospheric composition." The climatic parameters often associated with such changes are temperature, rainfall and humidity as well as others such as atmospheric particle pollution and wind. These primary changes are caused principally through an increase in greenhouse gas emission through the atmosphere.

There have been many forecasts of the effects of global warming, among which are melting of the polar ice caps and glaciers, rising sea levels, changes in weather patterns, fresh water shortages, climatic changes, coral reef bleaching and an increase in surface temperature. Patz and Kovats have listed six major areas of concern to human health in response to ongoing climatic change. They called it the "hotspots in climate change and human health". The list includes heat waves, rise in sea levels, flooding, drought, malnutrition, El Nino effects and highland malaria. However, others have argued that these are direct effects and therefore indirect effects should also be included. It has, therefore, been postulated that due to the rising global temperature more areas of the world would favor the survival of tropical insects such as mosquitoes. This would lead to the spread of these insects towards the northern and southern hemisphere as well as higher altitudes. Since it is known that mosquitoes act as vectors and are responsible for the transmission of diseases such as malaria, yellow fever and dengue fever, global warming can be viewed as a factor in the incidence of these diseases. Series of studies have attempted to correlate increased incidence of malaria to climatic change. A study by Gao et al. found that malaria incidence decreased in Auhui Province of China in the 1990s but that there was a significant increase in the north (the province had three regions: north, mid and south) since 2000 while transmission was relatively low in the middle and south. Using Spearman correlation, they found that the monthly incidence of malaria was significantly associated with temperature, rainfall, relative humidity and multivariate El Nino/

Southern Oscillation index with lags of 0-2 months in all three regions. Polynomial distributed lag (PDL) showed that rainfall within 1-2 months was associated with monthly incidence over a 2-year predictive period. They, therefore, concluded that changes in rainfall are associated with the re-emergence of malaria in the north Anhui Province. However, others have argued that there is no link between an increase in malaria incidence and climatic change. Reiter, in a review, argued that future changes in climate may alter the prevalence and incidence of malaria but he believed that the obsessive emphasis on global warming as a dominant parameter is indefensible. He, therefore, stated that the principle determinants are linked to ecological, societal, political and economical parameters. However, lessons learned on the ground would support the proponents of the view that "global warming plays a significant role in the increase of the incidence of malaria.

Treating Asymptomatic Carriers

Asymptomatic carriers of the parasite are known for not seeking any treatment for their infection. They, therefore, constitute a reservoir for the parasite resulting in public health risk. Systematic identification as well as treatment of these carriers can be used as one of the intervention strategies to reduce the parasite reservoirs. If these pools are reduced, it will have an impact on reducing the transmission of the parasite.

Intermittent Presumptive Treatment (IPT) in Pregnancy

This involves giving a curative treatment dose of an effective antimalarial drug to a pregnant woman at predefined intervals. It was initially introduced in high malaria transmission areas in order to reduce the adverse effect of *P falciparum* in pregnancy. However, based on the results of clinical trials which showed that IPT could reduce anemia in young children as well as malaria episodes, it was extended as a measure of reducing morbidity and mortality in the first year of life. Anti-chemoprophylaxis for pregnant women has been practiced for many years using chloroquine and pyrimethamine. However, due to the limitation of these drugs in preventing *P falciparum* malaria, sulphadoxine-pyrimethamine (SP) is now recommended as an alternative. With the reported increased in the incidence of resistance to SP, there is an urgent need to evaluate other options such as IPT. A treatment dose of SP (25mg sulfadoxine/1.25mg pyrimethamine per kilogram body weight) can last up to 60 days in cases of fully sensitive *P falciparum*, but dosing depends on full age or weight-adjusted treatment derived from either practical evidence or from dose dependent findings which, in most cases, involves non- pregnant women. The dose and timing interval should be determined by absorption, tolerability, distribution and the elimination kinetics of the drug used and the *in vivo* minimal inhibition concentration (MIC). It has been suggested that the ideal interval between doses should not be more than one week longer then the time required for plasma concentration to fall from peak post-dose levels to the MIC value. With increasing resistance to SP, is it ideal to use ACT for IPT? Jansen, in a commentary, argued that artesunate therapies including artesunate or artemether could be theoretically possible for IPT and represents a valid option to sulfonamide alone. Cisse et al. reported that there was a clear-cut prevention of malaria over a 13-week follow up period when they used a single dose of artesunate combined with a dose of SP. However, such a combination could be dangerous and may lead to the development of resistance since this combination is not capable of reducing the parasite load. The WHO recommends ACT as the first-line treatment of *P falciparum* malaria. This guideline states that artemisinin derivative should be used to treat uncomplicated *falciparum* malaria in the second and third trimester of pregnancy but should not be used in the first trimester unless they are the only treatment available or the patient's life is threatened or if treatment with clindamycin plus quinine has failed. Others have therefore suggested the use of a fixed combination of artesunate and sulphamethoxypyrazine (SMP). In addition, data has shown that when women are exposed to AL during the second and third trimester periods, it was well tolerated and no adverse outcome for the mother or her exposed fetus was observed. However, more safety data is required for the first trimester period.

Counterfeit Drugs

It is estimated that 700,000 people die as a result of fake TB and malaria drugs in developing countries. Counterfeit drugs in malaria control are a public health problem. Poor quality antimalaria drugs can have an adverse effect on the health outcome by failing to reduce the load of the parasite or delaying treatment with high quality drugs. A systematic review of 18 studies showed that untreated or inadequate treatment of *P falciparum* during childhood can have short and long-term neurocognitive consequences and through higher risk of anemia adversely have an impact on the cognitive development of the child. Inadequate antimalaria doses could increase drug resistance while when other drugs are added to the counterfeit drugs might mask important clinical signs and cause adverse effects. Counterfeit drugs are thought to make US$600 billion in worldwide trade. The WHO and various governments have recommended and implemented a series of measures to combat this menace but it keeps increasing. Several studies have attempted to provide data on the extent of the problem. A meta-analysis from 21 countries in Sub-Saharan Africa and 7 from Southeast Asia concluded that 32% of the tested samples failed a quality test. Bate also concluded that as much as 15% of the global drug supply outside the developed countries is counterfeit. What causes this counterfeiting? In Sub-Saharan Africa, a variety of causes has been postulated. According to the WHO, Africa countries lack the capacity to control the quality, safety and efficacy of the drugs in circulation on their markets or passing through their territories. Erhun et al. in a study also listed vested interest both on the part of the regulatory officials and counterfeiters as an important reason.

What should be done to counter this menace? First, there is the need to put in place an effective surveillance system, improve regulatory procedures and establish a simple tracking, reporting and information system. There is also the need to encourage good practice which encourages the process of good manufacturing practice with a strong post market surveillance system. The legal system should also be strengthened and those caught in the net should be tried as murderers. However, others have argued that such an action will drive the perpetrators underground resulting in armed conflict and corruption of regulatory officials. To achieve the optimal results, the international health regulations need to be invoked where new technologies that identify counterfeit drugs is the basis of such action.

Affordable Medicine Facility

If the stakeholders should advocate for malaria control without an affordable medicine program then the gain achieved will be lost. To prevent this, Affordable Medicine Facility –malaria (AMFm) was launched in 2004 with a bold idea as outlined in a U.S. Institute of Medicine (IOM) expert report:" Saving Lives, Buying Time: Economics of Malaria Drugs in Age of Resistance". The goal of this program was to subsidize the most effective antimalarial drugs at the top of the supply chain. The belief is that the drugs would then flow to patients as in the old order where older antimalarial drugs became available. The IOM made the following observations:

- ACT, the WHO-recommended first-line medicine for falciparum malaria is much more costly than their widely available competitors, now largely ineffective as a result of drug resistance.
- In Africa, antimalarial medicines are more likely to be purchased from private vendors than from public clinics which often have stock-outs
- Given the general inaffordability, minus subsidy, many shopkeepers would never stock ACT.

In 2008, the Global Fund assumed the financial and administrative procedures of AMFm but this was separated from the Fund's routine grant-making. A pilot involving seven countries was undertaken that was supported by the Roll Back Malaria Partnership, World Bank and other leading funders such as UNITAID, Bill & Melinda Gates Foundation and the UK International Department for Development. Under the pilot program, Ghana, as usual, received the first 'co-paid' ACT in August 2010 and the remaining countries came on board over an eight month period. An independent evaluation of the pilot reported that:

> 'Of the 8 pilots, success benchmarks were clearly met in 5 pilots for availability, 5 pilots for QAACT [Quality-assured artemisinin-combination therapy] price relative to the most popular antimalarial that is not a QAACT, and 4 pilots for QAACT market share. ... It is also possible that benchmarks were met in one additional pilot for availability and price, and in 3 additional pilots for market share, although the evidence is not as strong. ... The success benchmarks related to artemisinin monotherapy (AMT) price and market share were met in all pilots with sufficient AMT in the market to make these benchmarks relevant.'

The evaluators concluded that AMFm really changed the rule of the game by sending ACT to the villages. AMFm, as a result of the successful pilot, needs to be expanded. If this action is taken, more poor and vulnerable would be reached resulting in ACT coupled with RDTs to enable care givers to dispense antimalarial drugs to only those with proven malaria cases. This is in contrast to the prevailing situation where anybody with a febrile condition is given anti-malarial drugs. But taking into consideration the global financial crisis, another laudable project such as AMFm might be forced to either scale down or even close altogether. Defeating malaria requires multiple strategies as outlined in this chapter but such interventions should include easily accessible and effective drugs which are affordable. Some have called for ending user fees as done in Sierra Leone. A study in Mali showed that some of the respondent attributed user fees as a result of them seeking help from traditional healers and unregulated care givers. The WHO estimates that each year, healthcare costs push 100 million people into poverty. More studies need to be undertaken to better understand the effects of removing user fees. This would, in turn, inform future healthcare financing policy decisions.

Therefore, to continue making inroads, we must face reality and stop all the "hoping" agenda to more realistic ones which include expanding access to quality ACT for all who need them as well as developing new, potent and cheap antimalaria agents. For the advice to be given to the global community there is the need for perseverance with all control measures or the gains that have been made will surely be lost.

Malaria Funding

There has been significant improvement in the fight against malaria especially the Millennium Development Goal (MDG) of halting and reversing the incidence of malaria by 2015. This has resulted in countries such the United Arab Emirates, Morocco and Turkmenistan attaining the status of being malaria free between 2007 and 2012. Funding played a positive role in these achievements as there was a large increase in the available funds earmarked for malaria control. But funding for malaria control has reached a critical point. This can be attributed to the global financial meltdown and the subsequent austerity measures instituted by various governments around the world which has seen the reduction of funds. Commitments for future funding are becoming difficult to secure as the Global Fund to Fight Malaria, AIDS and Tuberculosis (Global Fund) have been forced to suspend new projects until2016 with a reduction of funding by US$500 in 2011 compared to 2010. In order to address this pressing issue, the Global Fund came up with a strategy "Investing for Impact". What this means is that the limited funds available would be deployed with maximum efficacy. What would be the best solution to this financial crisis? A look at the on the ground situation of Africa shows that funding is dominated by international support. Most Africa countries are control –focused with the majority of the projects funded by external donors. This has resulted in inequity driven by patterns in donor assistance. On the other land, countries with large governmental funding stand out in terms of equitable levels of funding, size of the population at risk or level of risk when compared to the rest of the region. Namibia and South Africa supported their elimination goal through domestic funding. An analysis by Pigott et al. found that in 2012, about US$2 billion of external funding was utilized for malaria control. This, when combined with national government funding, led to a total of US$2.5 billion spent in that year. However, the assessment suggested that the global malaria control effort required between US$4 to US$6 billion. What this means is there is a large deficit between what is needed and what is provided. There is the need to consider the malaria control needs as global and the challenge facing the global community is to increase the overall funding to a substantial level while consolidating the gains that have been funded over the past decade. There is no doubt that global funding for malaria control persists; there is the need to utilize all avenues to fill the gap. Critical analysis also shows that inequities exist and strategies must be developed to address them. The Global Fund's "Investing for Impact" should be regarded as the new principle for future funding whereby the most at risk- population will be targeted and disbursement of funds will be tailored to the needs while still framing funding decisions within the context of global disease contribution.

Insecticide Treated Net Beds (ITNS)

ITNS are one of the most effective preventive interventions against malaria infection and form the cornerstone of the Roll Back Malaria (RBM) Partnership's agenda of scaling up the impact of reducing malaria related mortality by 75% from 2000 to 2015. To achieve this target, RBM has set the target of reaching and sustaining 80% universal coverage with ITN, especially long lasting insecticide treated nets (LLINS). This means that 80% of all the population at risk of malaria should be sleeping under an ITN. The RBM strategic plan outlines that the 80% universal coverage target can be achieved using a combination of campaigns and continuous channels such as antenatal clinics (ANC) and expanded programs of immunization (EPI). The World Malaria Report of 2011 showed that 38 African countries had adopted the policy of ITN distribution through ANC, 79 through EPI and 36 through mass campaigns. Due to infrastructure challenges and equity concerns, most of the emphasis has been on mass campaigns through which hundreds of millions of ITNs has been distributed in Sub-Saharan Africa since 2002. In this regard, ITN can be view as a revolutionary tool which can be used to effectively control malaria. With ITN, there is little infringement of personal privacy and the application of insecticides does not involve seasonal upheavals of clothing and furniture. It also provides effective protection from the nightly nuisance of mosquitoes. However, it must be noted that untreated or improperly treated nets do not provide effective protection from mosquito bites. Therefore, it cannot be regarded as a means of personal protection as it is known that mosquitoes can feed through the net when body parts touch the net and access is also possible through small holes. The use of ITNs during pregnancy is associated with increased mean birth weight and a reduction in the risk of miscarriage or still births.

To sustain the success of the ITN program, there is the need for maximum effectiveness which can be achieved through delivering more ITNs using different channels. Equity should also be addressed as evidence has shown that the same children may be missed by all intervention due to low socioeconomic status or living in remote areas that maybe underserved even by mass campaigns. There has to be extensive coverage and the use of the bed nets is of great importance in achieving a significant reduction of malaria transmission as seen in the past with indoor sprays. The use of ITNs has now been integrated into national malaria control strategies. This should be encouraged. However, to attain optimal results, personnel involved in distributing the nets should be well enumerated. ITNs can replace indoor spray and it should be introduced in a systematic manner through a well informed strategy to the committed community. Public information is very essential and it must be taken as an ongoing activity.

Novel Vector Control

With the malaria vector becoming resistant to DDT, there is the urgent need to explore new strategies for controlling the vector. A study has shown that crushing the seeds of the neem tree (Figure 9) and sprinkling them on running or stagnant water has a killing effect on the vector. Neem seed kernel has insecticide properties as a result of a combination of about 99 compounds, with azadirachtin been the most potent with a concentration of about 5mg/g of kernel. The study showed that 2 weekly applications of neem powder to known breeding habitats of Anopheles resulted in an almost 49% reduction in adult female Anopheles Gambias s.l. mosquito in Baninzoumbon. This strategy can offer a long sustainable tool for the control of the malaria vector.

Other studies have shown the efficacy of use of neem kernels in the control of the larval stage of the vector. A study showed that exposing anopheline larvae to undiluted neem oil led to 100% mortality in 12 hours. Another study which used neem formulation on third and fourth stage of Anopheles gambiae s.i. larvae resulted in 50% inhibition of the emergence of adults at a concentration of 6ppm. However, it must be stated that resistance to neem-based compounds is more likely to rise as a result of refined larvicide which is based on a single compound than if the whole seed is used. The use of neem-based intervention also has some limitations: it is only directed against the larval stage and has no effect on adult mosquito. Therefore, the aim of such an intervention is to prevent the adult mosquito population from reaching large numbers. This is because once the adult populations are allowed to be established, the intervention will not be efficient. It has, therefore, been proposed that the most effective way of utilizing this intervention is applying the seed extract to breeding sites when the population is low during the dry season so that as many immature mosquitoes as possible can be eradicated thereby reducing the population available for breeding when the conditions becomes favorable. It has also been shown that the efficacy of seed extract degrades under sunlight after 7 days. This means it does not have much of an effect on the environment and constant application would be required to maintain efficacy.

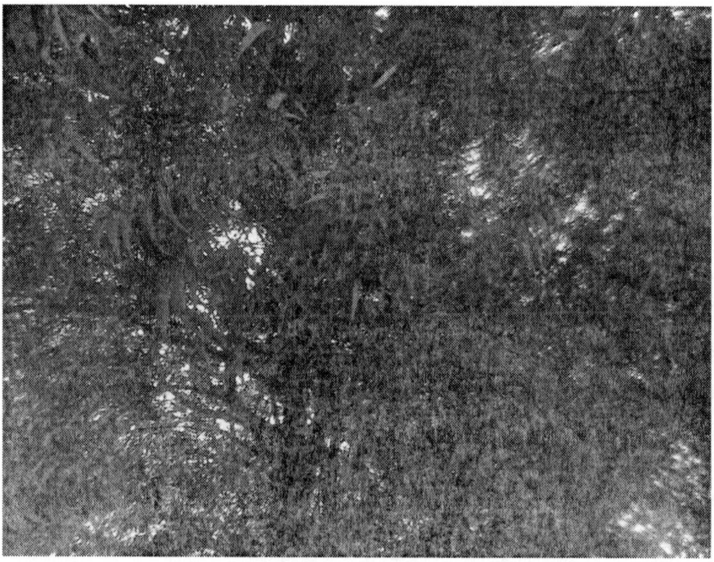

Figure 9. Neem tree in Kano State Nigeria.

Education

In the fight against malaria, we must take these factors into consideration: In Sub-Saharan Africa, where malaria is a major obstacle to social and economic development, it costs about US$12 billion lost every year in GDP. A challenge facing Africa is early diagnosis and treatment (EDT) of malaria before it becomes a complication. This involves all aspects of health behavior especially at the household level which includes home management of diseases and self-medication which is very rampant in this part of the world. Most of the antimalaria drugs used in the past are now of no use as explained earlier due to resistance. The world is now at the cross-roads because any resistance to ACT; the widely used antimalaria drug would be a catastrophic scenario. In spite of the numerous interventions that have been put in place so far, the malaria situation is still deteriorating. The obstacle to the success of these interventions can be linked to sociocultural, economic and political reasons. The WHO calls for the combination of ITNs and EDT in the RBM initiative with a recommendation of a control strategy comprising proper application of existing models as follows: EDTT of symptomatic malaria to prevent progression to severe and potentially fatal stages, preventive measures including the use of ITNs and selective residual spraying and prediction, containment and if possible prevention of epidemics as well as strengthening local capacities especially health care givers. However, in malaria control, local involvement is essential. Drug abuse which aids in the development of resistance is common across Africa and other risk areas. When the malaria vaccine is developed, the challenge stakeholders will face is acceptance. The polio vaccine is much aligned in some communities which is making eradication programs difficult. There is no doubt that polio is making a comeback. Supplying ITNs is not the issue but using it is. It will be no use if we accomplish the 70% target yet the people are not well informed to know the importance of using them. Therefore, any ideal control measure should include health education. A well informed community can play a significant role in the fight against malaria.

A study by Fataungase et al., had the objective of determining the effect of health education on the home management of malaria among caregivers of children under 5 years old in Ogun State Nigeria. It involved 1800 houses divided into experimental and control wards each made up of 200 respondents in which 180 of each group completed the questionnaire after a three month period. A training curriculum and program based on the health educational needs was developed and used for the experimental group. They found that knowledge of signs and symptoms of malaria was a statistically significant change in the control group. A similar result was obtained using home management of the malaria parameter. A significant important finding was the reduction in the reliance of herbs for home management of malaria which was linked to awareness created by the National Malaria Control Program and free distribution of antimalaria drugs. The association between training and the increased ability of the respondents to get the correct dose of the drug used, Malact® was also significant. No such relationship was observed in the control group that was not exposed to training. This study supports the argument that health education is essential. Schools also have a potential role to play in that they can reach a large portion of the population in a more effective and efficient way. They are very effective in disseminating information to children and their families in rural communities where access to information through mass media, literature and the internet is normally limited. A study in Tanzania involving school children reported that the primary sources of information on malaria was the school and teachers. In a study, it was recommended that there is the need to improve the content of textbooks on malaria. A study by Ataka et al. examining the possible factors of malaria prevalence concluded that information regarding lifestyles and attitudes toward bed net use as well as malaria education experience at school are particularly important for practical malaria prevention. Another study in Ethiopia supports the call that the effort to control malaria could be influenced by improving access to education especially for women. In addition, more initiative to improve education should target al.l group of travelers such as last-minute travelers, business travelers, those visiting friends, elderly travelers and solo-travelers.

The T3: Test. Treat. Track

On World Malaria Day 2012, Dr Margaret Chan, the WHO Director General launched a new initiative called T2: Test. Treat. Track with an appeal to malaria endemic countries, donors and the global community to scale up diagnostic testing, treatment and surveillance for malaria. This will be an ideal initiative for malaria endemic countries.

Human Factor

Despite the achievements attained in the global effort against malaria, it still remains an important public health issue with an estimated 3.3 billion people at risk globally while 655,000 deaths were associated with malaria in 2010. Human factors would play a crucial role in the continuous effort to control malaria. In most communities in Sub-Saharan Africa visited by this author, people were supplied with treated bed nets. However, most people do not use them while others use them irrationally. This results in the development of resistance to the bed net. A study in Tororo Uganda found that despite the provision of bed nets and prompt treatment with ACT, the incidence of malaria was very high and appeared to be on the rise which means there was the need to identify additional intervention strategies. What should be added is that although the authors did not include determination of resistance in their study, it is quite obvious that resistance was playing a part in the prevalence of malaria in Tororo. Therefore, addressing human behavior should be one of the novel interventions. Another important human factor is the building structure in communities at risk. Several studies have explained the impact of house structure on vector-borne diseases. In Senegal, a study reported that the initial successes of a treated bed net program were partially offset by an increase in insecticide resistance which resulted in a rebound of the incidence of malaria. In Tanzania it was also reported that the vector an arabiensi avoided ITNs. Data has proved that transmission of many vector-borne diseases is facilitated by housing design that favors the entry of mosquitoes. Subsequently, improving and screening of the house structure had a great impact on the control and elimination of the malaria vector in many richer countries. Several studies have presented data on various housing characteristics that favor mosquito entry. These include the presence of eave gaps, lack of ceilings and the lack of screening over windows and doors. In addition, a randomized control study has shown that blocking all potential house entry points for mosquitoes had a very great impact on mosquitoes, reduces vector densities and the entomological inoculation rate (EIR). A study in North Tanzania showed a strong association between houses, individuals and behavioral risk factors with malaria transmission. In their argument, the authors suggested that their finding needs to be complemented with entomological data for a better understanding of malaria transmission in human dwellings. A study by Lwetoijere et al. conducted in a high transmission setting to assess the impact of housing structure on malaria transmission, concluded that despite the significant reduction in vector density and malaria transmission as a result of large coverage of ITNs, high numbers of host-seeking malaria vectors were still found indoors due to the design of the houses which favors mosquito entry. Another important aspect is human behavior. The scientists and policy makers can devise some of the best control strategies but they will remain useless if the people do not change their dirty habits. By visting cities across Africa, it is possible to see that they provide an environment conducive for the vector to thrive.

From this and other data, it can be suggested that the various national public health institutions as well as building authorities need to get down to real business if the global malaria control programs are to be a success. A new novel Knowledge, Attitude and Practicing (KAP) strategy on malaria needs to be developed within the national context.

Controlling Imported Malaria

In the past it was postulated that together with drug resistance and unsustainable funding, human population movement (HPM) was regarded as among the important causes of failure in malaria control. These factors still remain threats. Human movement from high to low or non- malaria endemic areas can lead to the introduction of imported malaria thereby posing a challenge to the health system as well as ongoing transmission. Statistically, the influx of malaria-infected individuals determines the vulnerability of a population where each introduced imported case presents a risk of starting an outbreak. Understanding the paradox of HPM patterns would assist in developing novel strategies in evidence-based control of malaria as suggested by a study which postulated that human movement patterns should be factored in when decisions are to be taken regarding disease elimination and prevention. Imported malaria has been described to be one of the major risk factors in Zanzibar with the expansion of the road rail and air transport network implicated in the spread of vector-borne diseases through human and vector movement.

The World Health Organization referred this concept as "vulnerability" which is defined as "the frequent influx of infected individuals or groups and infective anophelines". The quantitative status of route of malaria importation includes all parasites that pass through boarder posts in human and vectors. This means the vulnerability a populace to imported malaria depends on an area's "receptivity" for malaria which is based on the condition of transmission "through the abundant existence of the vector anophelines and other ecological as well as climatic conditions". A paper outlined a mathematical model on how malaria can be imported into a community as follows: Human residents of a specific community can be become infected while traveling abroad then return home for the duration of the infections, human visitors can be spend some time in a community after being infected elsewhere, human immigrants infected somewhere and then move permanently into the community and finally an infected mosquito can travel into a community. Imported malaria should now be viewed as a global problem taking into consideration the swiftness of human and vector movement. In the United States, data showed that in 2008, 1,298 malaria cases were detected which were imported mainly by tourists who were inadequately protected. In the UK, it was found that between 1987 and 2007, 25,054 cases of falciparum malaria were detected in patients who had mostly traveled to Africa visiting friends and relatives. The data showed that the risk of malaria associated mortality is highest in the elderly, tourists and those presenting in areas where malaria is seldom seen. This means, pre-travel advice is quite essential. In Albania, since 1994, cases of malaria have been detected after it was thought to have been eradicated. One of the major risk factors associated with this reintroduction are migration movements and environmental factors such as flooding which changed the ecological equilibrium; although all the reported cases of malaria are imported.

Control of imported malaria should now be added to national control policies which should be based on multi-strategies aimed at stopping pathogen importation and preventing reintroduction. Therefore, chemoprophylaxis should be adequately prescribed to travelers. There should also be effective surveillance systems at points of entry which should include rapid diagnostic tests, provision of antimalaria drugs to those who failed to take some from their country of origin and an effective reporting system and vector control measures. A case study reported the first imported case of *P ovale* infection in Malaysia in 2010 which was initially misdiagnosed as *P vivax* infection.

Malaria Vaccine

Due to the ineffectiveness of malaria control strategies and increasingly burden of antimalarial drug resistance, the development of a malaria vaccine should be an urgent priority. The ideal vaccine should be cheap, safe, and able to induce life-long immunity, be active against all strains of the parasite and possess the ability of nearly complete interruption of the malaria life cycle through vaccine-induced immune response. Developing a malaria vaccine is hampered by some scientific and non-scientific challenges. The scientific challenges are: 1. Extensive genetic diversity in the candidate vaccine antigen. As has been seen in genetically diverse pathogens such as HIV, vaccines based on a polymorphic malaria protein might not induce responses against all the variants of the target antigen circulating in the parasite population. It could even result in an increased frequency of variants which are not targeted by the vaccine. This means that antigenic polymorphism is a difficult hurdle that must be overcome in the development of an effective malaria vaccine. For example, a single clone of the parasite has approximately 50 different copies of gene that code for the variable surface antigen PfEMP1. During chronic infection, each successive phase of parasitaemia express new variant surface antigens which allow the parasite to multiply despite the presence of antibodies directed against the previous parasitic wave; 2. The parasite possesses a complicated life cycle with different antigens expressed in each stage. Therefore, a vaccine effective in killing the parasite in the liver stage might not be able to inhibit the parasite in blood-stage 3. The parasite possesses a vast array of proteins which are estimated to total at least 5,000-6,000. This presents a very difficult choice for designing a subunit vaccine, 4. At the parasite-host interface, humans are known to exhibit unique heterogeneity in their immune response which is dependent on their type of human leukocyte antigen (HLA) and other factors. There is a wide array of other genetic traits such as hemoglobin type and red cell polymorphism that have an effect on the susceptibility and have been selected by malaria, 5. Scientists currently do not have an adequate understanding of the mechanism of the disease and the immunity or correlation of protection necessary for selection of the candidate which will proceed to clinical trials.

The non-scientific challenges include: 1. Inadequate funding, 2. Too little cooperation among scientists and funding agencies, 3. Mixed levels of interest from the developing countries, 4. Limited private sector participation and interest, 5. A knowledge of how to procure and distribute a successful vaccine, 6. Some have touted for a whole parasite approach. This may offer a high level of efficacy but may not be brought to the scale necessary to meet global demand for the vaccine and 7. The cost involved in the entire vaccine development process would be high driving potential manufacturers away from it.

However, there are several reasons to believe that malaria vaccines are biologically feasible. It has been found that people who are subjected to long-term malaria transmission develop some partial protective immune response to malaria. Immune people generally have fewer and less dense parasitaemia and are less likely to suffer clinical manifestations when parasiteamic. It has been reported that this immunity provides significant protection from malaria associated mortality. The immune protection includes antibody response which is involved in killing the erythrocytic stage of the parasite while transfer of immunoglobulin G to naïve human volunteers have been found to reduce *P falciparum* parasitemia by about 99%. A Malaria Vaccine Technology Roadmap has been created to explore how the key players in malaria vaccine development can work differently to accelerate the development of an effective malaria vaccine with the objective of developing a first generation vaccine by 2015 and a second generation vaccine by 2025.

Vaccine Design

Since evidence points to the fact that a malaria vaccine is possible, certain questions need to be answered including: what is the best strategy for designing the vaccine? What antigen should be used? How should it be formulated?

Vaccines contain several components each with a specific function. Synthetic peptides and purified recombinant protein vaccines' main objective is the induction of antibodies having one or more B-cell epitopes. T-cell epitopes are normally added to such vaccines to induce T-cell. These epitopes are then presented to the antigen-presenting cells (APC) in the delivery system. Vaccines have the intention of raising either the $CD4^+$ or $CD8^+$ cytotoxic lymphocyte (CTL) response containing one or more lymphocytes (T-cell epitopes, perhaps T-helper lymphocytes epitope and a delivery system which optimizes the interaction of the vaccine and the APC). Delivery systems are essential in vaccine strategies. Examples of delivery systems are aluminum hydroxide, live vectors such transfected live vaccinia and self-assembling lipids such as liposome. Specifically with the malaria vaccine what should be the guiding principle? The following is a summary of such guidelines:

- There is the need to choose antigens that meet the specific criteria.
- We should combine antigens from different stages of the parasite life cycle.
- We need to combine several antigens from a single stage of the parasite life cycle.
- There is the need to keep vaccines as simple as possible.
- The vaccine should induce the right kind of immune response.
- A functional and stable form of the antigen should be generated.

- We should have the ability to measure antimalaria immune effector function in vitro.

Vaccine Antigens

Several promising antigens of the parasite have been discovered from the life cycle of *Plasmodium* which is being explored as components of a potential malaria vaccine. Below is a brief description of some of them.

Pre-erythrocytic Antigen

Circumsporozoite protein (CS)

The CS protein is expressed on the surface of sporozoite in a large amount. It molecular weight (MW) varies depending on the species; for example *P berghei* has a MW of between 45 to 55 kDa while *P yoelii* and *P vivax* has MW of 65-75kDa and 40-66 kDa respectively. It has a central area of repeated amino acid sequences that have been found to be highly immunogenic and is present in all *Plasmodium* species. Monoclonal antibodies against these repeated regions of *P berghei*, *P yoelii* and *P vivax* have been reported to passively offer some protection when transferred to an animal previously challenged with infectious sporozoites. The repetition amino acid sequence found in *P falciparum* CS protein is made of asparagine-alanine-asparagine-proline (NANP). It has been used as an immunogen in some studies. For example, in a study it was shown that two of eleven vaccinated subjects were fully protected from sporozoite challenge. Another showed that passive transfer of cytotoxic $CD8^+$ T cells which recognized CS protein protected mice from challenge in *P berghei* and *P yeolii* murine malaria models. A study involving an immunized human with irradiated *P falciparum* showed the presence of $CD8^+$ and $CD4^+$ cytotoxic T cells that recognized a portion of the *P falciparum* CS protein. This evidence proved that a cytotoxic T-cell dependent antibody- independent protein which is based on immunity to the CS protein can be induced. This suggests that CS protein can be used as an excellent candidate for the development of a vaccine that has the ability of inducing both antibody and cell-mediated immunity.

SSP

This is a second sporozoite-associated protein which was identified on the surface of the sporozoite of the murine malaria parasite *P yoelii* and named sporozoite surface protein 2 (SSP2). When the transformed mouse cell expressing this protein was used in immunizing naïve mice, partial protection was induced. Similarly, when both SSP2 and CS protein expressing cells were used, all the mice were protected. The induced protection was $CD8^+$ T cell dependent. Transfer of the T-cell clone protected naïve animals.

Liver Stage Antigen 1 (LSA1)

LSA1 is a 230kDa protein which is expressed by infected hepatoctytes and contains about seventeen amino acid repeat. It has been shown that naturally exposed West Africans produced HLA-restricted cytotoxic. T cells that are able to recognize a 9 amino acid peptide from LSA1 in association with HLA Bw53. It has further been shown that the presence of HLA Bw53 correlated with protection against malaria. This suggests that immunity to LSA 1 might provide some form of protection against severe malaria.

Merozoite and Erythrocytic Antigen

Erythrocyte Binding Antigen 175 (EBA-175)

It is a 175 kDa protein that is expressed on the surface of merozoites and is thought to act as a ligand for attachment of merozoites to specific receptors on the erythrocytes. Its encoding gene has been sequenced. It has been found that part of the sequence encodes a B-cell epitope which when synthesized and used to immunize rabbits, the hyperserum at a 1:5 dilution is capable of reducing merozoites from invading the erythrocyte by about 80%.

Merozoite Surface Protein 1 (MSP 1)

This is a 195 kDa protein which is synthesized during the development of schizont. Some of its fragment is shed during invasion of the erythrocyte retaining 19 kDa fragment. This is found within a newly infected cell. It has been reported that immunization with *P falciparum* MSP 1 protects the *Samiri* and *Aotus* monkey. It has also been found that a 15 kDa recombinant subunit of *P yoelii* protected mice from lethal challenge.

MSP 2

Is a 45 kDa protein attached in the merozoites membrane and contains a central repeat region. There is sequence variation in about 50% of the protein, although the N and C-terminal regions are conserved.

Ring-infected erythrocyte surface antigen (RESA): It is also known as Pf155 and is a 155 kDa protein produced by *P falciparum* during late schizogony and expressed on the surface of an erythrocyte infected with ring stage parasite. RESA has a tandemly repeated amino acid sequence and the antibody from humans is reported to inhibit invasion of erythrocyte by merozoites in vitro.

Apical Membrane Antigen 1 (AMA1)

AMA 1 is a protein found on the organelle of merozoite and on the surface of merozoite. It consists of 546 amino acid residue in which three sub domains have been identified. The sub domains I, II, III are demarcated by a disulfide bond. Sequences of AMA 1 from *P falciparum* have been reported and analysis of these sequences showed that AMA 1 occurs as distinct allelic variants differing by the number of point mutations. In sub domain I, 41 polymorphic nucleotides and about 49 different nucleotide substitutions have been described. Of these, only 3 of the mutations are synonymous. Sub domaina II and III have only 9 polymorphic sites with no synonymous mutations. It has been reported that immunization with AMA 1 does induce antibodies that inhibit the parasite's invasion of merozoites thereby conferring some protection in the animal model.

Serine Repeat Antigen (SERA)

Is also known as serine protein 1 and p126 and is found within the parasitophorous vacuole. In *P falciparum*, its MW is 111 to 113 kDa. It has a serine content of 11% and data showed that the *Saimiri* monkey when immunized with SERA became protected from latter challenge of the infectious parasites.

Transmission-Blocking and Pathogenicity Antigen

Psf25

It is a 25 kDa protein which is found on the surface of *P falciparum* zygotes and ookinetes. It is one of the promising transmissions blocking vaccine immunogens. It was found that monoclonal antibody to Pfs25 blocks the transmission process by interfering with sexual stage development of the parasite within the mosquito.

Cytoadherence Antigen

Cytoadherence is mediated by several molecules which are expressed on the surface of infected erythrocyte to the vascular endothelial cells. One such molecule is Sequestrin, a 270 kDa protein expressed on the surface of infected erythrocyte. Also indentified is ligand CD 36, a recognition protein expressed by vascular endothelial. The variant parasite-derived protein (PfMP 1 var family) has also been identified on the surface of *P falciparum* infected erythrocyte.

Malaria Vaccine in Clinical Trials

As highlighted earlier, we do not currently have an effective malaria vaccine and it is not clear that a highly effective vaccine is in the pipeline. Many factors have been implicated including the scarcity of research funding. In recent years, global funding for malaria vaccine development has barely reached 25% of the approximately $684 million invested the development of an elusive HIV/AIDS vaccine. Other factors mentioned earlier in this book are the sheer complexity of the parasite and its complicated life cycle, extensive antigenic variations and the poor understanding of the interaction between *P falciparum* and the immune system. Aggravating the vaccine development efforts are the large gap in our understanding of *P falciparum* infection biology. These gaps can be closed only with adequate research support and the recruitment of experts in all facets of *P falciparum* immunology and biology. With increased funding, vaccinologists can broaden their scope of understanding and thereby increase the probability of success. So far, the strategies utilized are: pre-erythocytic vaccine, asexual stage vaccine, transmission-blocking vaccine and a combination of pre-erythrocytic and blood stage vaccines. A series of clinical studies have been and continue to be performed around the globe, of which four are analyzed below.

RTS, S Candidate

Will there ever be an effective malaria vaccine? RTS, S provides some hope for the world for it has consistently been shown to confer some partial protection against malaria and clinical malaria episodes in phase II studies. It is made of chimaeric recombinant protein which is expressed in *Saccharomyces cerevisiae*, comprising the central repeat and C terminal portion of the *P falciparum* CS protein and fused to Hepatits B virus surface antigen (HBs) combined in excess of HBs into a virus like particle. It is administered with an adjuvant ASO1 (Figure 10). When administered to Kenyan and Tanzanian children aged 5 to 17 months, it was found to be safe. It also reduced the risk of clinical *P falciparum* malaria by about 50% in the first 8 months after vaccination and about 45% over a period of 15 months. Most importantly, RTS, S is the first malaria to enter phase III clinical studies. It has been found to be associated with eliciting reaction to infection and CS-specific antibody titres and between resistance to clinical malaria, CS-specific interferon (IFN)-γ and secreted interleukin (IL)-2 responses but these correlations have not been associated with protection at the individual level.

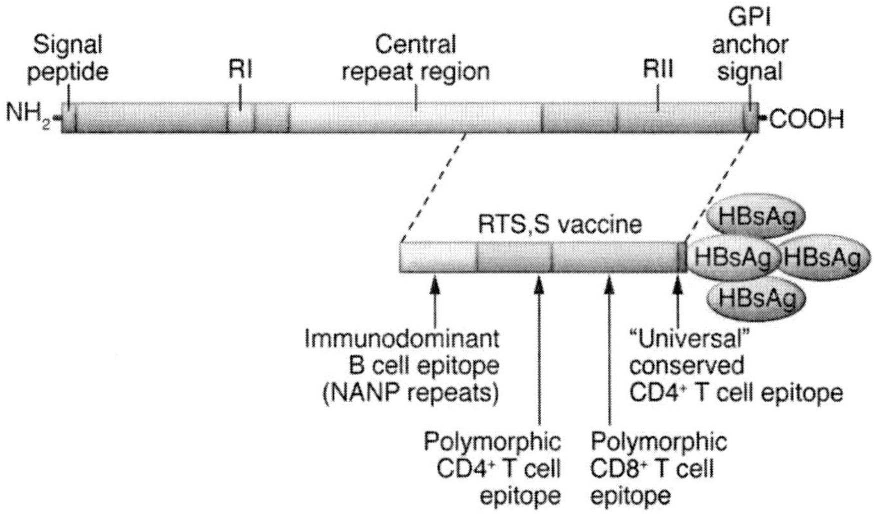

Figure 10. Schematic representation of the CSP and RTS, S vaccine. (Adopted from Crompton et al.)

A study by Horowitz et al. showed that RTS, S/ASO1 boosts the cellular response induced before HBV vaccination. This can be detected through the upregulation of CD69, CD15 and IFN-γ in CD4+ T cells, upregulation of CD69 and IFN-γ among NK cells and enhanced PBMC secretion of IL-2, IFN-γ and IL-40. In addition, RTS, S vaccination induces CD4+ T cell and NK cell response to CS peptide. A study by Olutu et al. found that RTS, S/ASO1E confers sustained efficacy for at least 15 months and shows promise as a potential public health intervention against childhood malaria in malaria endemic countries. However, further studies are required to establish the efficacy of the vaccine in children with HIV infection or those suffering from malnourishment. Other studies concluded that RTS, S is safe, well tolerated and immunogenic but its protection is short-live with a study showing that it confers protection for 14 months. RTS, S vaccine has been postulated to confer protection based on the manifestation of malaria. An exploratory study by Guinovart et al. to assess the difference in duration of protection to understand the protection afforded by RTS, S vaccine found that in the first cohort made of those with clinical malaria, efficacy against clinical malaria did not wane over time but in cohort 2 with infection, the efficacy decreased with time. They, therefore, proposed that reduced protection is due to early diagnosis and treatment of infection in cohorts which resulted in preventing exposure to asexual stage antigens. Long term protection associated with cohorts might be due to prolonged exposure to low-dose stage asexual parasitemia. A Phase III clinical study has shown that RTS, S vaccine provided 50% efficacy protection in young children and infants from clinical malaria up to 18 months after vaccination. Though half efficacy is not enough, it can be regarded as a major breakthrough. However, the study presented that the overall efficacy of the vaccine declined over a period of time in that previous results from the one year follow up of the phase III showed that the efficacy of the vaccine was 56% against clinical malaria and 47% against severe malaria for subjects aged 5-17 months old and 37% against severe malaria in subject aged 6-12 week old.

Clinical studies have outlined some adverse events associated with the RTS, S vaccine such as fever and local reaction. Despite its efficacy, RTS, S does not provide complete protection but reduces the risk of infection for each exposure. There are some challenges that need to be overcome if RTS, S vaccine is to become a success. These include the dosing schedule as a study reported that a second dose of RTS, S in volunteers resulted in generalized symptoms. The stability profile of the vaccine needs to be identified. The next challenge is what would be the final formulation of the vaccine. Finally, the most prominent challenge is how to send the vaccine to those who really need it after the pre and post-license bottlenecks.

MSP3-LSP Candidate

In an open randomized, 2- adjuvant Phase I clinical trial, Audra et al. evaluated the safety and immunogenicity of increased doses of a long synthetic peptide construct which spanned the conserved region of MSP3 targeted by biologically active antibodies (MSP3-LSP). The trial used 35 healthy volunteers who were randomized to receive three subcutaneous injections on day 0, 30 and 120. 100 injections were administered and 10 caused local reactions, 62 caused transient mild to moderate local reactions while 28 caused no reaction. No vaccine related serious adverse events were noticed through the trial. Montamide ISA 720 and aluminum hydroxide was the used adjuvants. They reported that MSP3-LSP vaccine was immunogenic with both adjuvants, although there was unacceptable reactogenic when it was combined with Montamide and concluded that the candidate vaccine had some benefit as it induced strong cytophilic response that are key agents of antibody-dependent, monocyte –mediated inhibition of the growth of the parasite. In a Phase 3 clinical study of RTS, S among African children, the authors concluded that it provided protection against both clinical and severe malaria in the recipients. However, no reduction in the rate of death from malaria or from any cause in the RTs, S/ASO1 group was observed. The authors postulated further that ASO1 provided protection against any existing disease and its associated deaths. In the older age group, the vaccine was more reactogenic than rabies vaccine in terms of both systemic and local effects. There was generalized convulsion during the 7 days after RTS, S/ASO1 vaccine at about 1 per 1000 vaccine doses.

MSP2-C1 Candidate

McCarthy et al. in dose escalating, double-blinded placebo-controlled phase I study in healthy malaria-naïve adults used MSP2-C1, a vaccine candidate containing recombinant forms of the two families of msp2 alleles, 3D7 and FC27 which was formulated in equal amounts with Montanide® ISA 720 as a water-in-oil emulsion found that majority of the subjected vaccinated with MSP2-C1 developed an antibody in response to both forms of MSP2. These antibodies mediated antibody-dependent cellular inhibition provided further call for MSP2 as a malaria vaccine candidate. However, the study showed that due to the reactogenicity of the formulation, further clinical development of MSP2-C1 requires formulation of MSP2 in an alternative adjuvant.

Plasmodium Vivax Vaccine Candidates: The burden of *P vivax* is increasing while the conventional methods used to control the spread of *vivax* malaria such as the use of drugs and bed nets are becoming ineffective. This makes it prudent for the international community to explore the prospect of developing an effective vaccine to reduce vivax associated malaria. Unlike the *P falciparum* vaccine development portfolio, *P vivax* vaccine development is just in Phase 1 clinical studies. This is attributed to some factors such as technical restrictions and lack of funding support. Lack of an efficient and continuous in vitro culture system has also impeded the development of vaccine candidates. Despite these difficulties, there have been some activities towards the development of a vaccine for *P vivax*. Several *P vivax* proteins which are homologous to *P falciparum* from different stages of the parasite's life cycle have been identified and two of these proteins, the CSP and Pvs25 have been tested in Phase 1 clinical studies. In 1987, a *P vivax* recombinant CSP (rPvCS-1) was targeted as a potential vaccine candidate after it was shown to induce high neutralizing antibodies in response to mice. It followed with two clinical trials using the recombinant protein but it did not induce significant immune response to enable the international community to develop it further. Another study also attempted to use a recombinant *P vivax* CSP which contained chimeric central repeat made of VK210 and VK247 produced in E coli. These were used for immunogenicity studies in mice. The recombinant CSP formulated in Montanide ISA 720, Montanide ISA 51 and incomplete Freund's adjuvants inoculated in BALB/c mice was shown to be highly immunogenic and induced antibodies that was able to agglutinate live sporozoites. Herrera et al. in a study aimed at testing the safety and immunogenicity of a vaccine made of *P vivax* CS-derived or synthetic protein N, R or C in a double blinded found that the vaccines were well tolerated and no serious AE were observed. The fragment of N and C had functional domains (RI and RII plus that has the ability of binding to hepatocyte ligands and involved in sporozoite invasion of the hepatocyte. The central repetitive domain is represented by peptide R which contains B-cell epitopes which is able to induce invasion-blocking antibodies. Herrera et al. showed that the peptides N and R elicited humoral response at dose 10, 30 and 100μg/dose. Antibodies to the three peptides recognized *P vivax* sporozoite in an immunoflourent antibody test. They concluded that the vaccine appeared to be safe, well tolerated and immunogenic in malaria- naïve volunteers. This is an encouraging result which provides hope for Phase II study. In addition, just like in *P falciparum*, some stage specific antigens have been targeted as potential vaccine candidates. These include sporozoite surface protein/trombospondin related adhesive protein (SSP2/TRAP), Duffy binding protein, MSP-1, AMA-1 as well as the Pvs25 and Pvs28.

Two Phase 1 clinical studies were conducted using Pvs25. In one of the studies, a dose-escalating strategy was utilized using a recombinant Pvs25 which was expressed in S cerevisiae and formulated with Alhydrogel®. The vaccine was called Pvs25H and found to induce antibodies which had transmission inhibiting properties. There was no serious AE. In the other study, the safety and immunogenicity of recombinant Pfs25 and Pvs25 formulated with Montanide ISA 51 was assessed. The formulation showed some transmission inhibiting activity but the trial had to be stopped after half of the volunteers developed local AE as well as a few systemic serious AE.

Conclusion: Future of Malaria

Where do we collectively go from the present in regards to malaria? There is no doubt that the world has chalked up significant progress in the fight against the malaria menace.

However, the future of malaria infection looks a bit murky in that we do not know what the future holds. The future of malaria infection depends on:

- Drug resistance: The future of malaria control hinges on how the burden of drug resistance is tackled. Among the future strategies to be facilitated are developing a pragmatic review of malaria policies to promote the rational use of antimalaria drugs and effective case management. A publicly accessible central database that contains information on the level of drug resistance also needs to be developed. In this way, data can be recorded in real time so that the data can be accessed, analyzed and used productively by all interested parties.
- Innovative laboratory diagnostic techniques: In the past, many malaria cases especially among children under the age of 5 years old, treatment was based on presumptive diagnosis using some lists of symptom, especially fever. The World Health Organization recommends that a diagnostic test should be performed for suspected malaria cases before treatment is initiated. But in some communities in Sub Saharan Africa, this is not adhered to. Efforts must be geared toward sensitization on this. With the assumption that malaria cases are dropping, there is a danger of over or misdiagnosis which might lead to an unnecessary and expensive treatment regimen. Failing to treat the underlying cause of the symptoms and presenting inaccurate malaria surveillance reports would result from such a danger. There is also the need to facilitate the development of basic laboratory tools and better rapid diagnostic kits which will be cost effective in the developing countries.
- Insect control: Insect control will continue to be an important aspect of any malaria infection control program. As outlined in this book, two interventions are currently being deployed: indoor residual spraying and long lasting insecticide treated beds which have been found to effective in reducing transmission. In order to have an effective system of control, there is the need to build up the capacity of those involved in malaria control programs so that the interventions being deployed can improve the scarce resources available while developing new interventions that are cost-effective and efficient. It has been recommended that in the future, a potential method which can be utilized is the use of a transgenic mosquito. In addition, the issue of insecticide resistance needs to be monitored closely.

- Vaccine: Developing a working and affordable malaria vaccine is now a priority but its development is faced with major challenges. Most of the efforts in the malaria vaccine development are targeted against *P falciparum*. Strategies need to incorporate the genetic diversity of both the parasite and human host as well as striving hard to develop effective immunity against the different stages of the parasite's life cycle. A vaccine against *P vivax* also needs to be tackled with urgency.
- Funding: Funding is crucial to malaria control but due to donor fatigue, all the gains made in the fight against malaria are being threatened. As a result of the recession, international donors and governments are tightening aid funds which have seen a significant reduction in aid to developing countries. What the developing countries need to know is that donor funding will not last forever. Therefore, there is the need to develop sustainable alternative funding which can fill the gap due to donor fatigue.
- The 5th *Plasmodium* species: In 2004, Singh et al. reported on a naturally-acquired *P knowlesi* infection from macaques in human beings after examining 208 people with malaria in Kapit division. The series of data has also highlighted the importance of *P knowlesi*-associated malaria infection in humans. Strategies need to be developed to include *P knowlesi* in clinical management of *Plasmodium*-associated disease.

Further Reading

Abate A, Degare A, Erko B (2013): Community knowledge, attitude and practice about malaria in a low endemic setting of Shewa Robit Town, northeastern Ethiopia; *BMC Public Health*, 13:312.

Abdullah, S., K. Adazu, H. Masanya, et al. (2007): Patterns of Age-Specific Mortality in Children in Endemic Areas of Sub-Sahara Africa; *Am J Trop Med hyg*, 77 (Suppl 6): 99-105.

Actian, J., AO Talisuna, et al. (2011): Quinine, an Old anti-malarial drug in a modern world: role in the treatment of malaria; *Malaria J*, 10:144.

Adama, I., D. Darko & S. Accorsi (2004): Malaria Burden; *Bulletin of Health Informatics*, 1:28-34.

Adam I et al. (2008): Artesunate plus sulphadoxine-pyrimethamine in the treatment of uncomplicated Plasmodium falciparum malaria during pregnancy; *Trans R Soc Trop Med Hyg*, 100:632-635.

Adjuik M et al. (2002): Amodiaquine-artesunate versus amodiaquine for uncomplicated Plasmodium falciparum malaria in African children: a randomized, multicenter trial; *Lancet*, 359:1365-72.

Agomo CO, Oyibo WA (2013): Factors associated with risk of malaria infection among pregnant women in Lagos, Nigeria; *Infect Dis Poverty*, 2:19 (Epub ahead of print)

Aguiar ACC, Santos RdM et al. (2012): Antimalaria activity and mechanisms of action of two novel 4-aminoquinolines against chloroquine-resistant parasites; *Plos One*, 7:e37259.

Allen, S. J. et al. (1999): Prevention of cerebral malaria in children in Papua New Guinea by Southeast Asian ovalocytosis band 3. *Am. J. Trop. Med. Hyg*. 60:1056-106.

Alifrangis M et al. (2009): Five-year surveillance of molecular markers of Plasmodium falciparum drug resistance in Konagwe District, Tanzania accumulation of 581G mutation in P. falciparum dihydropteroate synthetase gene; *Am J Trop Med Hyg*, 80:523-527.

Alin MH et al. (1996): Multiple dose pharmacokinetics of oral artemisinin and comparison of its efficacy with that of oral artesunate in falciparum malaria patients; *Trans R Soc Trop Med Hyg*, 90:61-65.

Alonso PL et al. (1991): The effect of insecticide-treated bed nets on mortality of Gambian children; *Lancet*, 337:1459-1502.

Alonso PL (2006): Malaria: deploying a candidate vaccine (RTS, S/AS02A) for an old scourge of human kind; *Int. Microbiol*, 9:83-93.

Alonso PL et al. (2011): A research agents to underpin malaria eradication; *Plos Med*, 8:e1000406.

Akachi Y & R Atun (2011): Effect of investment in malaria control on child mortality in Africa in 2002-2008; *Plos One*, 6:e21309.

Ajayi AA et al. (1998): Knowledge, attitude and practice of prednisolone prevention of chloroquine induced pruritus among Nigeria health workers; *Trop Doc*, 4:201-211.

Ancsin JB & Kisilevsky R (2004): A binding site for highly sulfated heparin sulfate is identified in the N terminus of the circumsporozoite protein; *J Biol Chem*, 279:21824-21832.

Andriantsoanirina V et al. (2011): In vitro susceptibility to pyrimethamine of DHFR 1164L single mutant Plasmodium falciparum; *Mal J*, 10:283.

Anthony MP et al. (2012): The global pipeline of new medicine in the control and elimination of malaria; *Mal J*, 11:316.

Anthony RL, et al. (1992): On-site diagnosis of Plasmodium falciparum, P. vivax, and P. malariae by using the quantitative buffy coat system. *J. Parasitol.* 78:994–998.

Anya SE (2004): Seasonal Variation in the risk and causes of maternal deaths in the Gambia: Malaria appears to be an important factor; *Am J Trop Med Hyg*, 70:510-513.

Armah HB, Wilson NO, Sarfo BY, Powell MD, Bond VC, et al. (2007): Cerebrospinal fluid and serum biomarkers of cerebral malaria mortality in Ghanaian children. *Malar J*, 6:147.

Arevalo-Herrera M et al. (1998): Mapping and comparison of the B-cell epitopes recognized on the Plasmodium vivax circumsporozoite protein by immune Colombians and immunized Aotus monkeys; *Ann Trop Med Parasitology*, 92:539-551.

Arevalo-Herrera M, et al. (2005): Immunogenicity and protective efficacy of recombinant vaccine based on the receptor binding domain of the

Plasmodium vivax Duffy binding protein in Aotus monkeys. *Am J Trop Med Hyg*; 73(5 Suppl):25-31.

Arrow K et al. (2004): *Saving Lives, Buying Time: Economics of Malaria Drug in an Age of Resistance.* Washington DC: The National Academies Press.

Ataka Y et al. (2011): Knowledge, Attitudes and Practices Relevant to malaria control in remote Island of Manus Papua Guinea; *Trop Med Health*, 39:109-117.

Askling, HH, Bruneel F, et al. (2012): Management of imported malaria in Europe; *Malaria J*, 11:328.

Awandare G.A. et al. (2007): Role of monocyte-acquired hemozoin in suppression of macrophage migration inhibitory factor in children with severe malarial anemia; *Infect Immun*, 75(1):201–10

Ayala E et al. (2006): Polymerase chain reaction and molecular genotyping to monitor parasitological response to anti-malarial chemotherapy in the Peruvian Amazon; *Am J Trop Med Hyg*, 74:546-55.

Babiker HA et al. (1994): Genetic evidence that R1 chloroquine resistance of Plasmodium falciparum is caused by recrudescence of resistant parasites. *Transactions of the Royal Society of Tropical Medicine and Hygiene* 88, 328–331.

Ballou WP et al. (1987): Safety and efficacy of a recombinant DNA Plasmodium falciparum sporozoite vaccine; *Lancet*, i: 1277-1281.

Ballou WR (2009): The development of the RTS,S malaria vaccine candidate: challenges and lessons; *Parasite Immunology*, 31:492-500.

Barnes KI, Durheim DN, et al. (2005): Effect of Artemether-lumefantrine policy and improved vector control of malaria burden in Kwa Zulu Natal South Africa; *Plos Med*, 2: e330.

Baruch DI et al. (1995): Cloning the P. falciparum gene encoding PfEMP1, a malarial variant antigen and adherence receptor on the surface of parasitized human erythrocytes. *Cell* 82: 77–87.

Baruch DI et al. (2002): Asexual blood stages of malaria antigen: Cytoadherence; *Chem Immunol*, 80:144-162.

Bartlett JMS, Stirling D (2003): A short history of the Polymerase Chain Reaction; *PCR Protocols*, 226:3-6.

BASCAP (2011): *Estimating the global economic and social input of counterfeiting and piracy*; Reports from the International Chamber of Commerce.

Bate R (2011): The market for inferior medicines: comparing the price of falsified and substandard products with legitimate medicine in emerging markets; *AEI Economic Policy Studies Working Paper*. 2011-05.

Bathurst I & Hentschel (2006): Medicines for malaria venture: sustaining antimalarial drug development; *Trends Parasitology*, 22:301-307.

Beare NAV et al. (2004): Prognostic significance and course of retinopathy in children with severe malaria. *Arch Ophthalmology*, 122:1141-1147.

Beare NAV et al. (2006): Malarial retinopathy: a newly established diagnostic sign in severe malaria. *Am J Trop Med Hyg*, 75:790-797.

Beier JC et al. (2008): Integrated vector management for malaria control; *Mal J*, 7 (Suppl 1):S4.

Bell D, et al. (2006): Emerging quality and access for malaria diagnosis: how can it be achieved? *Nar Rev Microbiol*, 4:682-695.

Bell D, et al. (2003): Making malaria testing relevant: beyond test purchase; *Trop Med Int. Health*, 8:876-883.

Ben MC et al. (2010): Targeting the lipid metabolic pathways for the treatment of malaria; *Drug Dev Res*, 71:44-55.

Bennett JW, Pyrus BS, Yadava A, et al. (2013): Primaquine failure and cytochrome P-450 2D6 in Plasmodium vivax malaria; *NEJM*, 319:1351-1352.

Bhattarai A, Ali S, et al. (2007): Impact of artemisinin-based combination therapy and insecticide-treated nets on malaria burden in Zanzibar; *Plos Med*, 4:e309.

Biagini GA et al. (2004): Generation of quinolone antimalarials targeting the Plasmodium falciparum mitochondrial respiratory chain for the treatment and prophylaxis of malaria; *PNAS*, 109: 8298-8303.

Binka F et al. (1996): Impact of perimethrin treated bednets on child mortality in Kasna Nankana district Ghana: a randomised controlled trial; *Trop Med Int. Health*, 1:147-154.

Birkholtz L-M, et al. (2012): Sustainable malaria control: transdisciplinary approaches for translational application; *Mal J*, 11:431.

Bisotti, Z, Marocco S et al. Acute intravascular haemolysis (black water fever) after malarial treatment. *Trop Med Int. Health*, 4:72-3.

Biswes AK et al. (2010): Increased financial accessibility and targeted education message could increase ownership and use of mosquito nets in Purulia District West Bengal India; *Trans R Soc Trop Med Hyg*, 104: 423-428

Black MJ et al. (1990): A single fragment of a malaria merozoites surface protein remains on the parasite during cell invasion and is the target of invasion-inhibiting antibodies; *J Exp Med*, 172:379-382.

Bobenchik AM, Witola WH, et al. (2013): Plasmodium falciparum phosphoethanolamine methyltransferase is essential for malaria transmission; *PNAS USA*, 110:18262-7.

Bodi JM, Nsibu CN, Longenge R, et al. (2013): Blackwater fever in Congolese children: a report of clinical, laboratory features and risk factors, *Mal J*, 12:205

Bojung KA et al. (2001): Efficacy of RTS, S/ASO2 malaria vaccine against Plasmodium falciparum infection in semi-immune adults men in the Gambia: a randomized trial; *Lancet*, 358:1927-1934.

Bozdech Z, Linas M, et al. (2003): The transcriptome of the intraerythrocytic developmental cycle of Plasmodium falciparum; *PLOS Biology*, 1:e5.

Brabin BJ, et al. (2001): An analysis of anemia and child mortality; *Nutr J*, 131(2S-2):636S–645S.

Brega S, Meshin B, et al. (2005): Identification of the Plasmodium vivax mdr-like gene (pvmdr1) and analysis of single-nucleotide polymorphism among isolates from different areas of endemicity; *J Infect Dis*, 191:271-277.

Breman JC et al. (2011): The role of research in viral diseases eradication and elimination programs: lesson for malaria eradication; *Plos Med*, 8:e1000405.

Brendts CH, et al. (1997): Effects of paracetamol on parasite clearance in Plasmodium falciparum malaria; *Lancet*, 350:704-709.

Bren C et al. (2011): Recent clinical and molecular insights into emerging artemisinin resistance in Plasmodium falciparum; *Curr Opin Infect Dis*, 24:570-577.

Breggs S, B Meslim, et al. (2005): Identification of the Plasmodium vivax mdr-like gene (pvmdr1) and analysis of single-nucleotide polymorphism among isolates from different areas of endemicity; *J Infect Dis*, 191:272-277.

Bridges DJ, Bunn J, et al. (2010): Rapid activation of endothelial cells enables Plasmodium falciparum adhesion to platelet decorated von Willebrand factor strings; *Blood*, 115:1472-1474.

Briolant S et al. (2012): Absence of association between piperaquine in vitro response and polymorphism in the *pfcrt, pfmdr1, pfmrp*, and *pfnhe* genes in Plasmodium falciparum; *Antimicrob Agents Chemother*, 54:3537-3544.

Bruce-Chwatt LJ (1974): Resurgence of malaria and its control; *J Trop med Hyg*, 77:s62-s66.

Bruce-Chwatt LJ (1987): Quinine and the mystery of black water fever; *Acta Leiden*, 55:781-96.

Bruce-Chwatt LJ (1987): Malaria and its control: Present situation and future prospects; *Ann Rev Public Health*, 8:75-110

Brunel F, Gachot B et al. Resurgence of black water fever in long-term Europeans in Africa: report of 21 cases and review. *Clin Infect Dis*, 32: 113-40

Beeson JG, Duffy PE (2005): The immunology and pathogenesis of malaria during pregnancy; *Curr Top Microbiol Immunol*, 297:187–227.

Brabin BJ (1983): An analysis of malaria in pregnancy in Africa; *Bull World Health Organ*, 61: 1005-1016.

Bradley J, Matias A, et al. (2012): Increased risk of malaria due to limited residual life of insecticide and outdoor biting versus protection by combined use of nets and indoor residual spraying in Bioko Isla; *Mal J*, 11:242.

Bray RS (1963): The malaria parasites of anthropoids apes; *Parasitol*, 49:888–891.

Breman JG (2004): Conquering the intolerable burden of malaria: what's new, what's needed: a summary. *Am J Trop med Hyg*, 71S2:1-15.

Brewster DR, Kwiatkowski DP, White NJ (1990): Neurological Sequelae of Cerebral Malaria in Children; *Lancet*, 336:1039-43.

Bruce MC, Donnelly CA, et al. (2000): Cross-species interactions between malaria parasites in humans; *Science*, 287:845–848.

Buffet PA, Gamain B, Scheidig C, Baruch D, et al.(1999): *Plasmodium falciparum* domain mediating adhesion to chondroitin sulphate A: a receptor for human placental infection; *Proc Natl Acad Sci U S A*, 96:12743–12748.

Butler, AR, Khan S, Ferguson E (2010): A brief history of malaria chemotherapy; *J R College Physicians Edinb*, 40:172-77.

Burn JM et al. (1989): A protective monoclonal antibody recognizes an epitope in the carboxyl-terminal cysteine-rich domain in the precursor of the major merozoites parasite of the rodent malaria parasite *Plasmodium yoelii; J Immunol*, 143:2670-2676.

Bzik DJ et al. (1992): Amino acid sequence of the serine-repeat antigen (SERA) of Plasmodium falciparum determined from cloned cDNA; *Mol Biochem*, 30:279-288.

Canfield CJ, et al. (1995): Interaction of atovaquone with other antimalarial drugs against Plasmodium falciparum *in vitro*; *Exp Parasitol*, 80:373-381.

Canadian International Development Agency (2000). *Canada announces $10 million to fight malaria in Africa*.

Cambron P et al. (2009): Development and technical and clinical validation of a qualitative enzyme-linked immunosorbet assay for the detection of human antibodies of recombinant hepatitis B virus vaccine; *Clin Vaccine Immunol*, 16:1236-1246.

Camus D & Hadley TJ (1985): A Plasmodium falciparum binds to host erythrocyte and merozoites; *Science*, 230:553-556.

Carrara VL, Sirilak S, et al. (2006): Deployment of early diagnosis and mefloquine-artesunate treatment of falciparum malaria in Thailand: the Tak Malaria Initiative; *Plos Med*, 3:e183.

Carter, R & Mendis KN (2002): Evolutionary and historical Aspects of the Burden of Malaria; *CMR*, 15:564-594

Casals-Pascual C. et al. (2006): Suppression of erythropoiesis in malarial anemia is associated with hemozoin in vitro and in vivo; *Blood*, 108(8):2569–77.

Casares S et al. (2010): The RTS,S Malaria vaccine; *Vaccine*, 28:4880-4894.

Cattamanchi A, Kyabayinze D, et al. (2003): Distinguishing recrudescence from reinfection in a longitudinal antimalarial drug efficacy study: comparison of results based on genotyping of msp-1, msp-2, and glurp; *Am J Trop med Hyg*, 68:133-139.

Carrar VI et al. (2009): Changes in the treatment response to artesunate-mefloquine in the northwestern border of Thailand during 15 years of continuous deployment; *Plos One*, 4:e4551.

Cattani JA, Gibson FD, et al. (1987): Hereditary ovalocytosis and reduced susceptibility to malaria in Papua New Guinea. *Trans. R. Soc. Trop. Med. Hyg*. 81:705-709

Cavalli-Sforza, L. L., P. Menozzi, and A. Piazza (1994): *The history and geography of human genes*. Princeton University Press, Princeton, N.J

Caufield L, et al. (2004): Undernutrition as an underlying cause of malaria morbidity and mortality; *Am J Trop med Hyg*, 71(Suppl 2): 55-63.

Ceesaay SJ et al. (2008): Changes in malaria incidence between 1999 and 2007 in The Gambia: a retrospective analysis; *Lancet*, 372:1545-1554.

CDC (1985): Adverse reaction to Fansider and update recommendation for its use in the prevention of malaria, *Morb Mortal Wkly Rep*, 8:713-714.

Chan-Ling T., Neill A. L., Hunt N. H. (1992): Early microvascular changes in murine cerebral malaria detected in retinal whole mounts. *Am. J. Pathol*. 140:1121–1130

Chansiri K., Phantana S (2002): A polymerase chain reaction assay for the survey of bancroftian filariasis. *Southeast Asian J. Trop. Med. Public Health* 33, 504–508.

Charman SA et al. (2011): Synthetic ozonide drug candidate OZ439 offers new hope for a single-dose cure on uncomplicated malaria; *PNAS*, 108:4400-4405.

Charoenvit Y., et al. (1987): Characterization of *Plasmodium yoelii* monoclonal antibodies against stage-specific sporozoite antigens; *Infect Immun*, 55:604-608.

Charoenvit Y et al. (1991): Inability of malaria vaccine to induce antibodies to a protective epitope with its sequence; *Science*, 251:668-671.

Charunwathana P et al. (2009): N-acetyl cysteine as adjunctive treatment in severe malaria: a randomized double-blinded placebo –controlled clinical trial; *Crit Care Med*, 37:516-527.

Chau Hong, T.T., Day NPJ, et al. (1996): Black water fever in Southern Vietnam: A prospective descriptive study of 50 cases, *CID*, 23:1274-81.

Checkley AM, et al. (2012): Risk factors for mortality from imported falciparum malaria in the United Kingdom over 20 years: an observation study; *BMJ*, 344:e2116.

Chenet SM et al. (2012): Genetic diversity and population structure of genes encoding vaccine candidate antigens of Plasmodium *vivax*; *Mal J*, 11:68

Chotivanich K, Udomsigpetch R, et al. (2012): *Plasmodium vivax* Adherence to Placental Glycosaminoglycan, *Plos One*; 7:e34509.

Chou M et al. (2012): Performance of "VIKIA Malaria Ag Pf/Pan" (IMACCESS®), a new malaria rapid diagnostic test for detection of symptomatic malaria infections; *Malaria J.*, 11:295.

Cinchona bark. [*http://historyofmalaria.com/2010/02/cinchona-bark/*].

Cisse B et al. (2006): Seasonal intermittent preventive treatment with artesunate and sulphadoxine-pyrimethamine for prevention of malaria in Senegalese children: a randomized placebo-controlled, double-blind trial; *Lancet*, 376:659-667.

Clark CJ, Haselden JN (2008): Metabolic profiling as a tool for understanding mechanism of toxicity; *Toxicol Pathol*, 36:140-147.

Coca SG, Parikh CR (2008): Urinary biomarkers for acute kidney injury: perspectives on translation; *Clin J Am Soc Nephrol*, 3:481–490.

Cohen J et al. (2012): Do patients adhere to over-the-counter Artemisinin Combination Therapy for malaria? Evidence from intervention study in Uganda; *Mal J*, 11:83.

Cohen JM et al. (2012): Malaria resurgence: a systematic review and assessment of its causes; *Mal J*, 11:122.

Cohen JM et al. (2012): Malaria resurgence: a systematic review and assessment of its causes; *Mal J*, 11:122.

Cohen S et al. (1961): Gamma-globulin and acquire immunity to human malaria; *Nature*, 192:733-737.

Cohn BA et al. (2007): DDT and breast cancer in young women: new data on the significance of age at exposure; *Environ Health Perspect*, 115:1406-1414.

Conroy AL, Phiri H, et al. (2010): Endothelium-Based Biomarkers Are Associated With Cerebral Malaria in Malawian Children: A Retrospective Case-Control Study; *Plos One*, 5(2): e15291. Doi:10.1371/journal.pone. 0015291.

Coppel RL et al. (1984): Immune sera recognize on erythrocyte a Plasmodium falciparum antigen composed of repeated amino acid sequences; *Nature*, 310:789-793.

Coppi A et al. (2005): The Plasmodium circumsporozoite protein is proteolytically processed during cell invasion; *J Exp Med*, 201:27-33.

Cosner C, et al. (2009): The effects of human movement on persistence of vector-borne diseases; *J Theor Biol*, 258:550-560.

Cramari A et al. (2007): Rapid microarray-based method for monitoring of all currently known single-nucleotide polymorphisms associated with parasite resistance to antimalaria drugs; *J Clin Microbiol*, 45:3685-3691.

Creasey AM, Staalsoe T, et al. (2003): Nonspecific immunoglobulin M binding and chondroitin sulfate A binding are linked phenotypes of Plasmodium falciparum isolates implicated in malaria during pregnancy; *Infect. Immun*, 71: 4767–4771.

Crompton PD et al. (2010): Advances and challenges in Malaria vaccine Development; *J Clin Inves*, 120: 4108-4178.

Crutcher J.M. et al. (1995): Interleukin-12 and malaria; *Research in Immunology*, 146:552–559.

Curtis CF & Mnzava AE (2000): Comparison of house spraying and insecticide – treated nets for malaria control; *Bull WHO*, 78:1389-1400.

Daly TM & Long CA (1993): A recombinant 15-kilodalton carboxyl-terminal fragment of *Plasmodium yoelii* 17XL merozoite surface protein 1 induce a protective immune response in mice; *Infect Immun*, 61:2462-2467.

Dame JB et al. (1984): Structure of the gene encoding the immunodominant surface antigen on the sporozoite of the human malaria parasite Plasmodium falciparum; *Science*, 225:593-599.

Daniel MC, Salanti A, et al. (2010) Igm, FcURs and Malarial Immune Evasion, *J Immunol*; 184:4597-4603.

Decuypere S et al. (2003): Pathogen genotyping in polyclonal infections: application of a flurogenic polymorphism chain reaction assay in malaria; *J Infect Dis*, 188:1245-1249.

Deen JL et al. (2001): The safety of the combination artesunate and pyrimethamine-sulfadoxine given during pregnancy; *Trans R Soc Trop Med Hyg*, 95:424-428.

De Monbrison et al. (2003): Real-time PCR for sensitivity assay and for pfmdr1-pfcrt single nucleotide polymorphism in Plasmodium falciparum; *J Microbial Methods*, 54:391-401.

Deitsch KW, del Pinal, A., and Wellems, T.E. (1999). Intra-cluster recombination and var transcription switches in the antigenic variation of Plasmodium falciparum. *Mol. Biochem. Parasitol.* 101:107–116.

Delacollete C, Cibanguka J et al. (1987): Compared response to chloroquinine, fansider, quinine, Quinidine slow release of infection with Plasmodium falciparum in the Kivu Region of Zaire; *Acta Leiden*, 55:159-165.

Deitsch KW, Calderwood MS, Wellems TE (2007): Cooperative silencing of var genes; *Nature*, 412:875-876.

Desakorn V, Silamut K, et al. (1997): Serum-quantitative measurement of Plasmodium falciparum antigen pfHRP-2 in blood and plasma; *Tredn R Soc Trop Med Hyg*, 91:479-483.

Diakite M et al. (2009): A genetic association study in The Gambia using tagging polymorphisms in the major histocompatibility complex (MHC) class III region implicates a HLA-B associated transcript 2 (BAT2) polymorphism in severe malaria susceptibility; *Hum Genet*, 125:105-109.

Djmde, A. et al. (2001): A molecular marker for chloroquine resistant falciparum malaria; *NEJM*, 344:257-263.

de Mast Q, Groot E, Lenting PJ, de Groot PG, McCall M, Sauerwein RW, Fijnheer R, van der Ven A (2007): Thrombocytopenia and release of activated von Willebrand factor during early Plasmodium falciparum malaria. *J Infect Dis*, 196:622-628.

Demirev PA, Feldman AB, et al. (2002): Detection of malaria parasites in blood by laser desorption mass spectrometry; *Anal. Chem*, 74:3262–3266.

Desai KR et al. (2010): Molecular modeling studies, synthesis and biological evaluation of derivatives of N-phenylbenzamides as Plasmodium falciparum dihyroorotate dehydrogenase (pfDHODH) inhibitors; *Medical Chemistry Research*, 20:321-332.

Dobson MJ (1994) Malaria in Europe: a geographical and historical perspective; *Parasitologia*, 36:35-60.

Donalson C (1990): Paying for publicly-Provided Goods: A possible measure of Benefit; *J Health of Economic*, 9:103-118.

Dondorp A, et al. (2005): Artesunate versus quinine for treatment of severe falciparum malaria: a randomized trial, *Lancet*; 366:717-725.

Dondorp AM et al. (2005): Estimation of the total parasite biomass in acute falciparum malaria from plasma PfHRP2; *Plos Med*, 2:e204.

Dondorp, A.M. & Day NP (2007): The treatment of severe malaria; *Trans R Soc Trop Med Hyg*, 101:633-634.

Dondorp AM et al. (2010): Artemisinin resistance: Current situation and scenario for containment; *Nat Rev Microbiol*, 8:272-280.

Dormer P, et al. (1983): Ineffective eryhtopoiesis in acute human P. falciparum malaria; *Blut*, 46(5):279–88.

Dorn A, et al. (1995): Malarial haemozoin/beta-haemozoin supports haem polymerization in the absence of protein; *Nature*, 374:269-271.

Doumbo OK et al. (2009): High levels of Plasmodium falciparum resetting in all clinical forms of severe malaria in African children; *Am J Trop med Hyg*, 81:987-993.

Draper CC and Sirr SS (1980): Serological investigations in retrospective diagnosis of malaria; *Br. Med. J*, 280:1575–1576.

Durand R et al. (2000): Use of molecular beacons to detect an antifolate resistance-associated mutation in Plasmodium falciparum; *Antimicrob Agents Chemother*, 44:3461-3464.

Duret L (2000): tRNA gene number and codon usage in the *C elegans* genomes are co-adapted for optimal translation of highly expressed genes; *Trends Genet*, 16:287-289.

Dutta S et al. (2007): Structural basis of antigenic escape of malaria; *PNAS*: 12488-12493.

Eastman RT & DA Fidock (2009): Artemisinin-based combination therapies: a vital tool in the effort to eliminate malaria; *Nat Microbiol*, 7:864-874.

Eastman RT, Pattaradilokrat S, et al. (2013): A class of tricyclic compounds blocking malaria parasite oocysts development and transmission; *AAC*, 57:425-435.

Egan JE et al. (1987): Efficacy of murine malaria sporozoites vaccines: implication for human vaccine development; *Science*, 236:453-456.

Ehrtardt S & Meyer CG (2009) Arthemeter-lumefantrine in the treatment of uncomplicated Plasmodium malaria; *Ther Clin Risk Manag*, 5:805-815.

Eibach D, Ceron N, et al. (2012): Therapeutic efficacy of arthermether-lumefantrine for Plasmodium vivax infection in a prospective study in Guyana; *Mal J*, 11:347.

Eisele TP et al. (2012): Estimates of child health deaths prevented from malaria prevention scale-up in Africa 2001-2010; *Mal J*, 11:93.

Enyati A & Hemingway J (2010): Malaria Management: Past, Present and Future; *Ann Rev of Entomology*, 55:569-591.

Escalante AA, Ayala FJ (1994) Phylogeny of malaria genus Plasmodium derived from rRNA gene sequence; *PNAS USA*, 91:11373-11377.

Eshetu T, Abdo N, et al. (2012) Open-label trial with artemether-lumefantrine against uncomplicated Plasmodium falciparum malaria three years after its broad introduction in Jimma zone, Ethiopia; *Malaria J*, 11:240.

Etard JF, Kodio B& Ronsmans C (2003) Seasonal variation in direct Obstetric mortality in rural Senegal: role of malaria? *American Journal of Tropical Medicine and Hygiene* 68, 503–504.

Etlinger HM et al. (1991): Ability of recombinant or native proteins to protect monkeys against heterologous challenge with Plasmodium falciparum; *Infect Immun*, 59:3498-3503.

Evans L (2012): Quality of anti-malarial collected in the private and informed sectors in Guyana and Suriname; *Mal J*, 11:203.

Falanga PB, Butcher E.C. (1991): Late treatment with Anti-LFA-1 (CD11a) antibody prevents cerebral malaria, *Microbe Infect*; 1:961-968.

Farnet A, Ursing J, et al. (2012). Artemether-lumefantrine treatment failure despite adequate lumefantrine day 7 concentrations in a traveler with Plasmodium falciparum malaria after returning from Tanzania; *Malaria J*, 11:176.

FDA (2008): Non clinical safety studies for the conduction of human clinical trials and market Authorization for pharmaceutical: FDA on *http://www/fda.gov/download/Regulatoryinform/Guidance/ucm129524.pdf* (Accessed on 02/11/2012).

Fields JW (1949): Blood exchange and prognosis in acute falciparum malaria; *Trans R Soc Trop Med Hyg*, 43:33-48.

Fiehu O, Kopka J, et al. (2000): Metabolites profiling for plant genomics; *Nat Biochem*, 18:1157-1161.

Files JC, et al. (1984): Automated erythrocyte exchange in fulminate falciparum malaria; *An Intern Med*, 100:396.

Fillinger U &Lindsay SW (2011): Larval source management for malaria control in Africa: myths and reality; *Mal J*, 10:352.

Final Report of the independent Evaluation of AMFm Phase 1: *http://www.theglobalfund.org/en/amfm/independentevaluation/*.

Findlay, GM & Stevenson AC (1944): Investigation in the chemotherapy of malaria in West Africa, Malaria suppression-Quinine & Mepacrine; *Ann Trop Med Parasitol*, 38:168-172.

Finley RW, Mackey LJ, Lambert PH (1982): Virulent P berghei malaria: prolonged survival and decreased cerebral pathology in T-cell-deficient mic; *J Immunol*, 129:2213-2218.

Flint J, Harding RM, et al. (1993): The population genetics of heamoglobinopathies; *Bailliere's Clin. Haematol*, 6:215-262

Florens LA, et al. (2002): A proteomic view of the Plasmodium falciparum life cycle; *Nature*, 419:520-526.

Foth BJ. et al. (2005): The malaria parasite Plasmodium falciparum has only one pyruvate dehydrogenase complex, which is located in the apicoplast; *Mol. Microbiol*, 55, 39–53.

Freitas-Junior LH, Hernandez-Rivas R, et al. (2005): Telomeric Heterochromatin Propagation and Histone Acetylation Control Mutually Exclusive Expression of Antigenic Variants Genes in Malaria Parasites; *Cell*, 121:25-36.

Fried M, Duffy PE (1996): Adherence of *Plasmodium falciparum* to chondroitin sulfate A in the human placenta; *Science*, 272: 1502-1504.

Fried M, Muga RO, Misore AO, Duffy PE (1998): Malaria elicits type 1 cytokines in the human placenta: IFN-gamma and TNF-alpha associated with pregnancy outcomes; *J Immunol*, 160: 2523-2530.

Fries LF et al. (1992): Liposomal malaria vaccine in humans: a safe and potent adjuvant strategy; *PNAS*, 89:358-362.

Galinski MR, Barnwell JW (2008): Plasmodium vivax: who cares? *Mal J* 7 (Suppl 1): S9.

Gallup JL & Sachs JD (2001): The economic burden of malaria; *Am J Trop med Hyg*; 64 (Suppl 1-2): 85-96.

Gamain B, et al. (1996): Increase in glutathione peroxidase activity in malaria parasite after selenium supplementation; *Free Radic Biol*, 21:559-565.

Gamble C et al. (2007): Insecticide-treated nets for the prevention of malaria in pregnancy: a systematic review of randomized control trial; *Plos Med*, 4:e107.

Gamo FJ et al. (2010): Thousand of chemical starting points for antimalarial lead identification; *Nature*, 465: 305-310.

Gao H-W et al. (2012): Changes in Rainfall Drives Malaria Re-Emergence in Anhui Province, China; *Plos One*, 7:e43686.

Garcia I, Araki K, Miyazaki Y, et al. (1995): Transgenic mice expressing soluble TNF-R1-IgG3 molecules are protected from lethal septic shock and cerebral malaria, and are highly sensitive to Listeria monocytogenes and Leishmania major infections. *Eur. J. Immunol.* 25:2401–2407.

Gardner MJ et al. (2002): Genome sequence of the human malaria parasite Plasmodium falciparum; *Nature*, 419:498-511.

Garett L (2012): Global health hits crisis; *Nature*, 482:7.

Gargano N, Ubben D, et al. (2012): Therapeutic efficacy and safety of dihydroartemisinin-piperaquine versus artesunate-mefloquine in uncomplicated Plasmodium falciparum malaria in India; *Malaria J*, 11:23.

Garley AE, Ivanovich E, et al. (2013): Gender difference in the use of insecticide –treated nets after a universal free distribution campaign in Kano State, Nigeria: post-campaign survey results; *Mal J*, 12:19.

Gary M, Gopinathan N, et al. (1990):Vivax malaria resistant to chloroquine: case reports from Bombay; *Trans R Soc Trop Med Hyg*, 12:656-657.

Gay F et al. (1996): Direct acridine orange fluorescence examination of blood slides compared to current techniques for malaria diagnosis. *Trans. R. Soc. Trop. Med. Hyg*. 90:516–518.

Gelpi AP, King MC (1976): Duffy blood group and malaria; *Science*, 191:1284.

Genton BF, Al-Yaman CS, et al. (1995): Ovalocytosis and cerebral malaria; *Nature*, 378: 564-565.

German PI & FT Aweeka (1998): Clinical Pharmacology of artemisinin-based combination therapies; *Clin Pharmokinet*, 47:91-102.

Gesase S et al. (2009): High resistance of Plasmodium falciparum to sulphadoxine/pyrimethamine in northern Tanzania and emergence of dhps resistance mutation at condon 58; *Plos One*, 4:e4569.

Gething PW, Patil AP, et al. (2011): A new world malaria map: Plasmodium falciparum endemicity in 2010; *Mal J*, 10:378.

Ghumra A, et al. (2008): Identification of residues in the Cmu4 domain of polymeric IgM essential for interaction with Plasmodium falciparum erythrocyte membrane protein 1 (PfEMP1); *J. Immunol*, 181: 1988–2000.

Gilles HM, Fletcher KM, et al. (1967): Glucose 6 phosphate dehydrogenase deficiency, sickling and malaria in African children in South Western Nigeria; *Lancet*, i: 138-140.

Global Fund to Fight AIDS, Tuberculosis and Malaria. Commitments and disbursements. [Accessed August 1, 2012]. 2009 *http://www.theglobal fund.org/en/commitmentsdisbursements/*

Gobbi F, Audagnotto S, et al. (2005): Blackwater fever in children in Burundi; *Emerging Infect Dis*, 11:1118-1120.

Goman M, et al. (1982): The establishment of genomic DNA libraries for the human malaria parasite *Plasmodium falciparum* and identification of individual clones by hybridisation. *Mol. Biochem. Parasitol.* 5, 391–400.

Gomes MF et al. (2009): Pre-referral rectal artesunate to prevent death and disability in severe malaria: a placebo-controlled trial; *Lancet*, 373:551-566.

Goodage R (2007): Metabolomics of super organism; *J Nutr*, 137:2595-2665.

Good MF (2005): Vaccine induced immunity to malaria parasites and the need for novel strategies, *Immunoparasitology*; 29-34.

Grad DJ, et al. (2013): Membrane active chelators as novel anti-African trypanosome and anti-malarial drugs; *Parasitol Int*, 62:461-463.

Graham IA et al. (2010): The genetic map of *Artemisa annua* L identifies loci affecting yield of the antimalarial drug artemisinin; *Science*, 327:328-331.

Grau G. E., Fajardo L. F., Piguet P. F., et al.(1987) Tumor necrosis factor (cachectin) as an essential mediator in murine cerebral malaria. *Science* 237:1210–1212

Grau GE, Pointaire P, Piguet PF, et al. (1991): Late administration of monoclonal antibody to leukocyte function-antigen 1 abrogates incipient murine cerebral malaria; *Eur J Immunol*, 21:2265–2267

Grau GE, Piguet PF, Enger D, et al. (1986): L3T4+ T lymphocytes play a major role in the pathogenesis of murine cerebral malaria. *J. Immunol.* 137:2348–235.

Graz B et al. (2008): Sublingual sugar for hypoglycemia in children with severe malaria: a pilot clinical study; *Mal J*, 7:242.

Grosnier C, Bustamante LY, et al. (2011): Basiginis is a receptor essential for erythrocyte invasion by Plasmodium falciparum; *Nature*, 460:534-537.

Guerin-Marchand C et al. (1987): A liver-stage-specific antigens of Plasmodium falciparum characterized by gene cloning; *Nature*, 329:160-164.

Guignemde WA et al. (2010): Chemical genetics of Plasmodium falciparum; *Nature*, 465:311-315.

Guinovart C, et al. (2009): Insights into Long-Lasting Protection Induced by RTS, S/ASO2A Malaria Vaccine: Further Results from a Phase IIb Trial in Mozambican Children; *Plos One*, 4: e5165.

Guyatt HL, et al. (2004): Use of intermittent presumptive treatment and insecticide treated bed nets by pregnant women in four Kenyan districts; *Trop Med Int Health*, 9:255-261.

Hadley TJ & Peiper SC (1997): From malaria to chemokine receptor: the emerging physiologic role of the Duffy blood group antigen, *Blood*; 89:3077-91.

Hadtsch M (2004): Quality and reliability of current malaria diagnostic methods, *Travel Med Infect Dis*; 2:149-160.

Hamel MJ et al. (2008): Dihydrofolate reductase 1164L mutation in Plasmodium falciparum isolates: Clinical outcome of 14 Kenya adults infected with parasites harbouring the 1164L mutation; *Trans R Soc Trop Med Hyg*, 102:338-345.

Hamer DH, et al. (2007): Improved diagnostic testing and malaria treatment practices in Zambia. *JAMA* 297: 2227–2231.

Hance P et al. (2005): Rapid immunochromatographic tests for detection of malaria: principles and strategies for use; *Med Trop*, 65:389-393.

Hargreaves K et al. (2000): *Anopheles furestus* resistance to pyrethroid insecticide in South Africa; *Med Vet Entomol*, 14:181-189.

Harris P et al. (2011): Automated erythrocytapheresis for severe malaria; *Intern Med J*, 41:60-63.

Hashimoto M et al. (1999): Genetic contribution of the BAT2 gene microsatellite polymorphism to the age-at-onset of insulin dependent diabetes mellitus; *Hum Genet*, 105:197-199.

Hanson KK, Ressurreicao AS, Bucholz K, et al. (2013): Torins are potent antimalarials that block replenishment of Plasmodium liver stages parasitophorous vacuole membrane proteins; *PNAS Early Edition*, www.pnas.org/cgi/doi/10.1073/pnas.1306097110

Hastings MD et al. (2002): Highly pyrimethamine-resistant alleles of dihydrofolate reductase in isolate of Plasmodium falciparum from Tanzania; *Trans R. Soc Trop Med Hyg*, 96:674-676.

Hastings MD, et al. (2004): The origin of antimalarial drug resistance; *Trends in Parasitology*, 20:512-518.

Hasting MD, Porter KM, et al. (2004): Dihydrofolate reductase mutation in Plasmodium vivax from Indonesia and therapeutic response to sulfadoxine plus pyrimethamine; *J Infect Dis*, 189:744-50.

Hastings IM et al. (2007): Molecular markers as indicators of antimalarial drug failure rates; *Trop Med Int Health*, 12:1298-1301.

Hawkins VN, Joshi H, et al. (2007): Antifolate can have a role in the treatment of Plasmodium vivax; *Trends Parasitol*, 23:213-22.

Hastings IM (2011): How artemisinin –containing combination therapies slow the spread of antimalarial drug resistance; *Trends Parasitol*, 27:67-72.

Haynes RK (2001): Artemisinin and derivative: the future for malaria treatment? *Curr Opin Infect Dis*, 14:719-726.

Hazra BR, Chowdhury RS, et al. (1998): Changing scenario of malaria: a study at Calcutta; *Indian J of Malariology*, 35:111-116.

Hedstrim RC et al. (1990): A malaria sporozoite surface antigen distinct from the circumsporozoite protein; *Bull WHO*, 68 (suppl1):152-157.

Herrera S et al. (2008): Safety and elicitation of humoral and cellular responses in Colombian malaria-naïve volunteers by Plasmodium vivax circumsporozoite protein-derived synthetic vaccine; *Am J Trop med Hyg*, 75 (Suppl 5): 3-9.

Herrington DA et al. (1987): Safety and immunogenicity in man of a synthetic peptide malaria vaccine against Plasmodium falciparum sporozoite; *Nature*, 328:257-259.

Hien TT et al. (1991): Comparative effectiveness of artemisinin suppositories and oral quinine in children with acute falciparum malaria; *Trans R Soc Trop Med Hyg*, 85: 210-211.

Hien TT (1994): An overview of the clinical use of artemisinin and its derivatives in the treatment of falciparum malaria in Vietnam; *Trans R Soc Trop Med Hyg*, 88 (Suppl 1): S7-S8.

Hill AVS, Catherine EM, et al. (1991): Common West African HLA antigens are associated with protection against severe malaria; *Nature*, 352:595-600.

Hirayasu K et al. (2012): Significant association of KIR2DL3-HLA-C1 combination with cerebral malaria and implication for co-evolution og KIR and HLA; *Plos Pathog*, 8:e1002565.

Holder AA & Freeman RR (1982): Biosynthesis and processing of a Plasmodium falciparum schizont antigen recognized by immune serum and monoclonal antibody; *I Exp Med*, 156:1528-1538.

Holding PA, Snow RW (2001): Impact of Plasmodium falciparum malaria on performance and learning: review of the evidence. *Am J Trop med Hyg*.

Horowitz A et al. (2012): Antigen-specific IL-2 secretion correlated with NK cells response after immunization of Tanzanian children with RTS, S/ASO1 malaria vaccine; *J Immunol*, 188:5054-5062.

Horton R et al. (2008): Variation analysis and gene annotation of eight MHC haplotypes: the MHC Haplotype project; *Immunogenetics*, 60:1-18.

Horuk, R., C. E. Chitnis, W. C. Darbonne, T. J. Colby, A. Rybicki, T. J. Hadley, and L. H. Miller (1993): A receptor for the malaria parasite Plasmodium vivax: the erythrocyte chemokine receptor. *Science* 261:1182-1184.

Howard RJ, et al. (1909): *Malaria and Greek history*, Manchester University Press; Manchester U.K.

Howard RJ, Uni S, et al. (1986): Secretion of a malaria histidine-rich protein (pfHRP II) from Plasmodium falciparum; *J Cell Biol*, 103:1269-1277.

Huang F. et al. (2012): Molecular epidemiology of drug resistance markers of Plasmodium falciparum in Yunnan Province, China, *Malaria J*; 11:243.

Heumekers M et al. (2012): Evaluation of the malaria rapid diagnostic test SDFK90: detection of both PfHRP2 and Pf-pLDH; *Mal J*, 11:359.

Hulka BS. *Overview of biological markers. In: Biological markers in epidemiology* (Hulka BS, Griffith JD, Wilcosky TC, eds), pp 3–15. New York: Oxford University Press, 1990

Hutagalung R et al. (2000): Influence of hemoglobin E trait on the antimalarial effect of artemisinin derivatives. *J. Infect. Dis*. 81: 1513-1516

Holmerg V, Onkamo P, et al. (2012): Mutation of complement lectin pathway genes MBL2 and MASP2 associated with placental malaria; *Malaria J*, 11:61

Hsu Y-H, Coleman JL & Tang WC (2011): Surface Morphological changes as biomarkers for detecting malaria infected avian erythrocyte, *Proceedings of 2011 International Conference on Micro technologies in Medicine and Biology* Lucerne Switzerland 4-6 May 2011.

Hwang J et al. (2010): Knowledge of malaria and its association with malaria-related behaviours-Results from the malaria indicator survey, Ethiopia 2007; *Plos One*, 5:e11692.

Hyunil J et al. (2012): Development of α-Helical Calpain Probes by mimicking natural protein-protein Interaction; *J Am Chem Soc*, 134:17704.

Idro R, Jenkins NE, Newton CRJ (2005): Pathogenesis, clinical features, and neurological outcome of cerebral malaria; *Lancet Neurol*, 4:827-40;

Idro R, Carter JA, Fegan G, Neville BG, Newton CRJ.Risk (2006): factors for persisting neurological and cognitive impairments following cerebral malaria; *Arch Dis Child*, 91:142-8.

IMACESS: *www.imacess.org* (Accessed on 28/11/12).

Iremenam NC et al. (2012): Temporal trends of sulphadoxine/ pyrimethamine (SP) drug-resistance molecular markers in Plasmodium falciparum parasite from pregnant women in Western Kenya; *Malaria J*, 11:134.

Jagannathan P, Muhindo MK, et al. (2012): Increasing incidence of malaria in children despite insecticide-treated bed nets and prompt anti-malarial therapy in Tororo Uganda; *Mal J*, 11:435.

Jain V, Armah HB, Tongren JE, Ned RM, Wilson NO, et al. (2008): Plasma IP-10, apoptotic and angiogenic factors associated with fatal cerebral malaria in India; *Mal J*, 7:83.

Jambon R et al. (2011): Pitfalls in new artemisinin-containing antimalarial drug development; *Trends in Parasitol*, 27: 82-90.

Jansen FH (2011): Intermittent preventive therapy for malaria: arguments in favour of artesunate and sulphamethoxypyraxine –pyrimethamine combination; *Mal J*, 10:70.

Jarolim, et al. (1991): Deletion in erythrocyte band 3 gene in malaria-resistant Southeast Asian ovalocytosis. *Proc. Natl. Acad. Sci. USA* 88:11022-11026.

Jatya Kumar DVR, Krisha D, et al. (2004): Impact of different house structure on filarial transmission in rural areas of Southern India; *South East Asia J Trop Med Public Health*, 35:587-590.

Jimoh A et al. (2007): *Quantifying the economic burden of malaria in Nigeria using the willingness to pay approach; Cost effectiveness and resource allocation*, 5:6. doi:10.1186/1478-7547-5-6

Joel G et al. (2004): Conquering the intolerable burden of malaria: what's new, what's needed: A summary; *Am J Trop med Hyg*, 71 (Suppl 2): 1-15.

Johnson A, et al. (2012): Hidden costs: The direct and indirect impact of user fees on access to malaria treatment and primary care in Mali, *Social Science and Medicine*, 75:1786-1792.

Jones C & Williams H (2004): The social burden of malaria: what are we measuring? *Am J Trop med Hyg*, 71: (Suppl 2): 156-161.

Jones TR & SL Hoffman (1994): Malaria vaccine development; *Clin Microbiol Rev*, 73:303.

Kaddurah-Daouk R, et al. (2008): Metabolomics: a global biochemical approach to drug response and diseases; *Ann Rev Pharmacol Toxicol*, 48:653-683.

Kakkilaya BS (2003): Rapid Diagnosis of Malaria; *Lab Medicine*, 34:602-608.

Kamau E et al. (2012): Development of a TaqMan Allelic Discrimination Assay for detection of single nucleotide polymorphism associated with antimalarial drug resistance; *Mal J*, 11:23.

Kamchowangpaison S & Meshnick SR (1996): The mode of action of the antimalarial artemisinin and its derivatives; *General Pharmacol*, 27:587-592.

Karbwang, J and NJ White (1990): Clinical Pharmacokinetics of mefloquine; *Clin Pharmacokinet*, 19:264-279.

Karmans W et al. (2002): Childhood growth and exposure to dichlorodiphenyl dichloroethane and polychlorinated biphenyls; *J pediatr*, 140:33-39.

Kazember LN, Kleinschmidt L & BL Sharp (2006): Patterns of malaria-related hospital admissions and mortality among Malawian children: en example of spatial modeling of hospital register data; *Malaria J*, 5:93.

Katinka, M.D., et al. (2001): Genome sequence and gene compaction of the eukaryote parasite Encephalitozoon cuniculi; *Nature*, 414:450-453.

Keiser J et al. (2005): Reducing the burden of malaria in different eco-epidemiological setting a with environmental management: a systematic review; *Lancet Infect Dis*, 5:695-708.

Kell DB (2007): Metabolomic biomarkers: search, discovery and validation; *Expert Rev Mol Dign*, 7:329-333.

Kelly J and J Trowsdale (2005): Features of MHC and NK gene clusters; *Transplant Immunity*, 14:129-135.

Kernoff LM et al. (1997): Exchange transfusion in sickle cell diseases using continuous flow blood separator; *Transfusion*, 17:269-271.

Kester KE et al. (2007): A phase I/IIa safety, immunogenicity, and efficacy bridging randomized study of a two-dose regimen of liquid and lyophilized formulation of the candidate malaria vaccine RTS, S /ASO2A in malaria-naïve adults; *Vaccine*, 25:5359-5366.

Kester KE et al. (2009): Phase 2a trial of 0,9 and 3 month and 0,7 and 28 day immunization schedule of malaria vaccine RTS, S/ASO2 in malaria-naïve adults safety, efficacy and immunologic associates of protection; *J Infect Dis*, 200:337-346.

Khattak AK, Venkatesan M, et al. (2013): Prevalence and patterns of antifolate and chloroquine drug resistant markers in Plasmodium vivax across Pakistan; *Mal J*, 12:310.

Khusmith S et al. (1994): Complete protection against Plasmodium yeolii by adopting transfer of a CD8+ cytotoxic T-cell clone recognizing sporozoite surface protein 2; *Infect Immun*, 62:2979-2983.

Kihara M et al. (2006): The effect of Plasmodium falciparum on cognition: a systematic review; *Trop Med & Int. Health*, 11:386-297.

Kitau J, Oxborough RM, et al. (2012): Species shifts in the *Anopheles gambiae* complex: Can LLINS successfully control *Anopheles arabiensis*? *Plos One*, 7: e31481.

Kleinschmidt I, Sharp B, et al. (2006): Reduction in infection with *P. falciparum* one year after the introduction of malaria control interventions on Bioko Island; Equatorial Guinea. *Am J Trop med Hyg*, 74:976-978.

Knapp B et al. (1989): Molecular cloning, genomic structure and localization in a blood stage antigen of Plasmodium falciparum characterization by a serine stretch; *Mol Biochem Parasitol*, 32:73-84.

Kochar DKP, Singh P, et al. (2003): Malarial hepatitis; *J Assoc Physician India*, 51:1069-1072.

Kochar DKP, Agarwal SK, et al. (2003): Hepatocyte dysfunction and hepatic encephalopathy in Plasmodium falciparum malaria; *QJM*, 96:505-512.

Kokwaro G. (2002): Ongoing challenges in the management of malaria; *Mal J* 8 (Suppl 1):S2.

Krishna S. et al. (2001): Bioavailability and preliminary efficacy of intrarectal artesunate in Ghana children with moderate malaria; *Antimicrob Agents Chemother*, 45:509-516.

Krishna S. et al. (2004): Artemisinin: Mechanisms of action and potential for resistance; *Drug Resistance Update*, 7:233-244.

Kurth F. et al. (2011): Pyronaridine-artesunate combination therapy for the treatment of malaria; *Curr Opin Infect Dis*, 24:564-569.

Kyes SA, Kraemer SM, and Smith JD (2007): Antigenic variation in Plasmodium falciparum: gene organization and regulation of the var multigene family; *Eukaryot. Cell*, 6: 1511–1520.

Kidson C (1992): Global malaria challenge: the Amsterdam summit Southeast; *Asian J Trop Med Public Health*, 23:635–40.

Kilian AH, Metzger WG, et al. (2000): Reliability of malaria microscopy in epidemiological studies: results of quality control; *Trop. Med. Int. Health*, 5:3–8.

Kiszewski A., Mellinger A, et al. (2004): A global index representing the stability of malaria transmission; *Am J Trop med Hyg*,70:486-498.

Kleinschmidt I., Schwabe C, Benavente L, et al. (2009): Marked increase in child survival after four years of intensive malaria control; *Am J Trop med Hyg*,80:882–88.

Kraemer SM and Smith JD (2006): A family affair: var genes, PfEMP1 binding, and malaria disease; *Curr Opin Microbiol*, 9: 374–380.

Kraisin S, Naka I, et al. (2011): Association of ADAMTS13 polymorphism with cerebral malaria; *Malaria J*, 10:366.

Kremsner PG, et al. (20090; Prognostic value of circulating pigmented cells in African children with malaria; *J Infect Dis*, 199(1):142–50

Kustner HG (1979): Trends in Four major communicable diseases; *S Afr Med J*, 58:460-73.

Kute VB, Trivedi HI, et al. 2012. Plasmodium vivax-associated acute kidney injury, India, 2010-2011, *Emerg Infect Dis*; 18:842-5.

Kwiatkowski D, Molyneux ME, et al. (1993) Response to monoclonal anti-TNF antibody in children with cerebral malaria; *Q. J. Med*, 86:91–98

Kyabayinze DJ, Karamagi C, et al. (2008): Multiplicity of Plasmodium falciparum infection predicts antimalarial treatment outcome in Ugandan children; *Af Health Serv*, 8:200-205.

Kyabayinze DJ et al. (2011): Operational accuracy and comparative persistent antigenicity of HRP2 rapid diagnostic test for Plasmodium falciparum malaria in a hyperendemic region of Uganda; *Mal J*, 7:221.

Larkin D, et al. (2009): Severe Plasmodium falciparum malaria is associated with circulating ultra-large von Willebrand multimers and ADAMTS13 inhibition. *PLoS Pathog*.

Laloo DG et al. (2007): UK malaria treatment guideline; *J Infect Dis*, 54:111-121.

Lalvani A et al. (1999): Potent induction of focuses Th-1 type cellular and humoral immune response by RTS,S/SBAS2, a recombinant Plasmodium falciparum malaria vaccine; *J Infect Dis*, 180:1656-1664.

Lamphier MS et al. (2006): TLR9 and the recognition of self and non-self nucleic acid; *Ann NY Acad Sci*, 1082:31-43.

Langhorne J et al. (2008): Immunity to malaria: more question than answers; *Nat Immunol*, 9:725-732.

Lewiery K, Ould Mohamed Salim Boukhary A, et al. (2012): Molecular surveillance of drug resistant Plasmodium vivax using pvdhr, pvdhps and pvmdr1 markers in Nouakchatt, Mauritania; *J Antimicrob Chemother*, 67:367-74.

Le Menach A, Tatem AJ, et al. (2011): Travel risk, malaria importation and malaria transmission in Zanzibar; *Science Rep*, 1:93.

Lengeler C (2004): Insecticide-treated bed nets and curtains for preventing malaria; *Cochrane Database Syst Rev*; 2:CD000363.

Leonardi E et al. (2001): Severe allergic reaction to oral artesunate: a report of tow cases; *Trans R Soc Trop Med Hyg*, 95: 182-183.

Levy GG, Nichols WC, et al. (2001): Mutations in a member of the ADAMTS gene family cause thrombotic thrombocytopenic purpura; *Nature*, 413:488-494.

Lim Y AL, Mahmud R, et al. (2010): Plasmodium ovale infection in Malaysia: first imported case; *Mal J*, 9:272.

Lindsay SW, Snow RW (1988): The trouble with eaves, house entry by vector of malaria; *Trans R Soc Trop Med*, 82:645-646.

Lindsay SW, Emerson PM, Charlwood JD (2002): Reducing malaria by mosquito protecting homes; *Trends Parasitol*, 18:510-514.

Lievens M et al. (2011): Statistical methodology for the evaluation of vaccine efficacy in a Phase III multi-centre trial of the RTS,S/ASO1 malaria vaccine; *Mal J*, 10:222.

Li GQ et al. (1994): Clinical trends of artemisinin and its derivatives in the treatment of malaria in China; *Trans R Soc Trop Med Hyg*, 88 (Suppl 1): S5-S6.

Li Q, et al. (2007): Pharmacokinetics and Pharmacodynamic profiles of rapid-acting artemisinin in the antimalarial therapy; *Current Drug Therapy*, 2:210-223.

Livingstone FB (1971): Malaria and human polymorphisms; *Ann. Rev. Genet*, 5:33-64.

Longnecker MP et al. (2005): Maternal serum levels of DDT metabolite DDE in relation to fetal loss in previous pregnancies; *Environ Res*, 97:127-133.

Loooareesuwan S, Wilairatana P, et al. (1999): Efficacy and safety of atovaquone/proguanil compared with mefloquine for treatment of acute Plasmodium falciparum malaria in Thailand; *Am J Trop med Hyg*, 60:526-32.

Lyke KE et al. (2011): Association of HLA alleles with Plasmodium falciparum severity in Malian children; *Tissue Antigen*, 77:562-571.

Lynch C et al. (2008): Emergence of a *dhfr* mutation conferring high-level drug resistance in Plasmodium falciparum population from Southwest Uganda; *J Infect Dis*, 197:1598-1604.

Lynn A, Chandra S, et al. (1999): Heme binding and polymerization by Plasmodium falciparum histidine rich protein II: influence by pH on activity and confirmation; *FEBS Lett*, 459:267-271.

Lasonder, E., et al. (2002): Analysis of Plasmodium falciparum proteome by high-accuracy mass spectrometry; *Nature*, 419:537-542.

Liu W, Li Y, Learn GH, et al. (2010): Origin of the human malaria parasite Plasmodium falciparum in gorillas; *Nature*, 467:420–425.

Livingstone FB (1971): Malaria and human polymorphisms; *Ann Rev Genet*, 5:33-64.

Lwetoijera DW, Kiware SS, et al. (2013): A need for better housing to further reduce indoor malaria transmission in areas with high bed net coverage; *Parasit Vector*, 6:57.

Lysenko AJA, Beljaev AE. An analysis of the geographical distribution of *Plasmodium ovale. Bulletin of the World Health Organization*, 1969, 40:383–394.

MacRae JI, Dixon MWA, et al. (2013): Mitochondrial metabolism of sexual and asexual blood stages of the malaria parasite Plasmodium falciparum; *BMC Biology*, 11:67

Madrid DC et al. (2008): Plasmodium falciparum purine nucleoside phosphorylase is critical for viability of malaria parasites; *J Biol Chem*, 283: 35899-35907.

Macallan DC et al. (2000): Red cell exchange erythrocytapheresis, in the treatment of malaria with high parasitaemia in returning travelers; *Trans R Soc Med Hyg*, 94:353-356.

MacCormark CP (1984): Human etiology and behaviour in malaria control in tropical Africa; *Bull World Health Organ*, 62 (Supp): 81-87..

Macgraith, J, Dorta de Mazzonelli G, et al. (1986): Clinical manifestation of malaria; *Clinics in Tropical Medicine & Communicable Diseases*, 1:127-170.

McCarthy JS et al. (2011): A phase 1 trial of MSP2-C1, a Blood –stage malaria vaccine containing 2 isoforms of MSP2 Formulated with Montanide® ISA 720; *Plos One*, 6:e24413.

McGregor IA et al. (1963): Treatment of East African P. falciparum malaria with West African human gammaglobulin; *Trans R Soc Trop Med Hyg*, 57:170-175.

Mahakur, A.C., Panda SN, et al. (1983): Malaria Acute Renal Failure; *J Assoc Phys India*, 31:613-616.

Maitland K, Williams TN & Newbold CI (1997) Plasmodium vivax and P. falciparum: biological interactions and the possibility of cross-species immunity. *Parasitology Today* 13, 227–231.

Makler, M. T., R. C. Piper, and W. Milhous (1998): Lactate dehydrogenase and diagnosis of malaria; *Parasitol, Today* 14: 376–377.

Mal ERA (2011): A research agenda for malaria eradication: vector control; *Plos Med*, 8: e1000401.

Malik A et al. (1991): Human cytotoxic T lymphocyte against the Plasmodium falciparum circumsporozoite protein; *PNAS*, 88:3300-3304.

Mali S, et al. (2008): Malaria surveillance- United States; *MMWR Surveillance Summ*, 59:1-15.

Manoj, T.D., T.S. Voss, A.J. Marty et al. (2005): Heterochromatin Silencing and Locus Repositioning Linked to Regulation of Virulence Genes in Plasmodium Falciparum; *Cell*, 121:13-24.

Marfurt J et al. (2001):The usefulness of twenty-four molecular markers in predicting treatment outcome with combination therapy of amodiaquine plus sulphadoxine-pyrimethamine against falciparum malaria in Papua New Guinea; *Mal J*, 7:61.

Marfurt J, de Monbrison F, et al. (2008): Molecular markers of in vivo Plasmodium vivax resistance to amodiaquine plus sulfadoxine-pyrimethamine: mutation in pvdhfr and pvmdr1; *J Infect Dis*, 198:409-417.

Marsh, K., Forster D, et al. (1995): Indicators of life threatening malaria in Africa children; *NEJM*, 332: 1399-1404.

Martens P, Hall L (2000): Malaria on the move: human population movement and malaria transmission; *Science Reports*, 1:93.

Mark K (2002): Artemisinin for severe malaria in Africa; *East Afri Med J*, 29:619-620.

Marsh K (1998): Malaria disaster in Africa; *Lancet*, 352:924

Mason, S. J et al. (1977): The Duffy blood group determinants: their role in the susceptibility of human and animal erythrocytes to Plasmodium knowlesi malaria. *Br. J. Haematol.* 36:327-335.

Matthews H, Usman-Idris M, et al. (2013): Drug repositioning as a route to anti-malarial drug discovery: Preliminary investigation of the in vitro anti-malarial efficacy of emetine dihydrochloride hydrate; *Mal J*, 12:359.

May J et al. (1999): HLA Class II factors associated with Plasmodium falciparum merozoites surface antigen allele families; *J Infect Dis*, 179: 1042-1045.

May J et al. (2001): HLA-DQB1*0501-restricted Th1 type immune response to Plasmodium Falciparum liver stage antigen I protein against malaria anemia and reinfection; *J Infect Dis*, 183:168-172.

Mayxay M, Pukittayakamee, et al. (2001): Persistence of Plasmodium falciparum HRP-2 in successfully treated acute falciparum malaria; *Trans R Soc Trop Med Hyg*, 95:179-182.

Meier, B. et al. (1992): Stage-specific expression of aldolase isoenzymes in the rodent malaria parasite *Plasmodium bergei. Mol. Biochem. Parasitol.* 52:15–27.

Meligy N (2007): The quest to be free of malaria; *Bull World Health Organ*, 85: 507-508.

Meshnick SR et al. (1996): Artemisinin and the antimalarial endoperoxide: from herbal remedy to targeted chemotherapy; *Microbiol Rev*, 60:301-315.

Milner DA, et al. (2005): Sampling of supraorbital brain tissue after death: improving on the clinical diagnosis of cerebral malaria. *J Infect Dis*, 191:805-808.

MMV (2012): Coartem Dispersible: www.mmv.org/achievements-challenges/ achievements/ coartem.d

MMV (2012): Target Product Profile on *www.mmv.org*

Moszynski P (2011): Global Fund suspends new projects until 2014 because of lack of funding; *BMJ*, 343:d7755.

Mout R et al. (2012): Anti-malarial activity of geldanamycin derivatives in mice infected with *Plasmodium yoelii*; *Mal J*, 11:54

Murray CJL et al. (2012): Global malaria mortality between 1980 and 2010: a systematic analysis; *Lancet*, 379:413-431.

McGlynn KA et al. (2006): Serum concentrations of 1,1,1-trichloro-2,2-bis (p-chlorphenyl) ethans (DDT) and 1,1-dichloro-2,2-bis (p-chlorophenyl) ethylene (DDE) and risk of primary liver cancer; *J Natl Cancer Inst*, 98:1005-1010.

McGlynn KA et al. (2008): Persistent organochlorine pesticides and risk of testicular germ cell tumor; *J Natl Cancer Inst*, 100:663-671.

Mechnick SR (2002): Artemisinin: mechanism of action, resistance and toxicity; *Int J Parasitol*, 32:1655-1660.

Meister S et al. (2011): Imaging of Plasmodium liver stage to drive next-generation antimalarial drug discovery; *Science*, 334: 1372-1377.

Meremikwu M & AG Marson (2002): Routine anticonvulents for treating cerebral malaria; *Cochrane Database Syst Rev*, 2: CD002152.

Miller LH, et al. (1975): Erythrocyte receptors for (Plasmodium knowlesi) malaria: Duffy blood group determinants; *Science*, 189:561-3.

Miller LH, et al. (1976): The resistance factor to Plasmodium vivax in blacks. The Duffy-blood group genotype, FyFy; *N Engl J Med*, 1976; 295:302-4.

Miller LH (1999): Evolution of the human genome under selective pressure from malaria: application for control; *Parassitologia*, 41:77-82.

Miller KD et al. (1989): Treatment of severe malaria in the United State with continuous infusion of huanidine gluconate and exchange transfusion; *NEJM*, 321:65-70.

Milner DA, Vareta J, Valim C (2012): Human cerebral malaria and Plasmodium falciparum genotypes in Malaria, *Malaria Journal;* 11:35.

Mishra SK, Mohanty S, et al. (1992): Hepatitis changes in plasmodium falciparum malaria; *India J Malariol*, 29:1167-1171.

Mishra S et al. (2012): Determinant of metabolic profile of antimalarial trioxane CDR1 99/411 in a rat liver microsomes using HPLC; *Biomed Chromatogr*, 26:115-122.

Mitrofanova A, Kleinberg S, et al. (2010): Predicting malaria interactome classification from true course transcriptomic data along the intraerythrocytic developed cycle; *Artif Int Med*, 49:167-176.

Mizuno Y, Kato Y, et al. (2009): First case of treatment failure of arthemether-lumefantrine in a Japanese traveler with imported falciparum malaria. *Jpn J Infect Dis*, 62:139-141.

Modiano D, Luoni G, et al. (2001): Haemoglobin C protects against clinical Plasmodium falciparum malaria. *Nature* 414:305-308.

Moonasar D et al. (2012): Malaria control in South Africa 2000-2010: beyond MDG 6; *Mal J*, 11:294.

Mohammed H et al. (2012): Paracheck-pf® Test versus Microscopy in the Diagnosis of Falciparum malaria in Arbaminch Zuri Woreda of South Ethiopia; *Ethiopia J Health*, 22:93-98.

Moorthy VS & Ballou WR (2009): Immunological mechanism underlying protection mediated by RTS,S: a review of the available data; *Mal J*, 8:312.

Moran M (2009): G-FINDER Neglected Diseases Research & Development: New Times, New Trends. Health Policy Division, The George Institute for International Health on *www.thegeorgeinstitute.org* (Accessed 8th January 2013)

Mordmuller B & PG Kremsner (1998): Hyperparasitaemia and blood exchange transfusion for treatment of children with falciparum malaria; *Clin Infect Dis*, 26:850-852.

Moreno A et al. (1991): Cytotoxic CD4+ T cells from sporozoite immunized volunteer recognize the Plasmodium falciparum CS protein; *Int. Immunol*, 3:997-1003.

Moriyama EN, Powell JR (1997): Condon usage bias and tRNA in Drosophila; *J Mol Evol*, 45:514-523.

Mota MM & Rodriguez A (2002): Invasion of mammalian host cells by Plasmodium sporozoites; *Bioassay*, 24:149-156.

Muhindo HM et al. 2012: Accuracy of malaria rapid diagnosis test Optimal-IT® in Kinshasa, the Democratic Republic of Congo; *Mal J*, 11:224.

Mullan F & S Frehywot (2007): Non-physician clinicians in 47 Sub Saharan African countries; *Lancet*, 370:2158-2163.

Nair S et al. (2002): Rapid genotyping of loci involved in antifolate drug resistance in Plasmodium falciparum by primer extension; *Int J. Parasitol*, 32:852-858.

Najera JA et al. (1998): *Malaria epidemic: detection and control, forecasting and prevention; Division of Control of Tropical Diseases*, World Health Organization.

Najera JA, et al. (2011): Some lessons for the future from the Global Malaria eradication Programme (1955-1969); *Plos Med*, 8:e1000412.

Navaratnam V. et al. (2000): Pharmacokinetics of artemisinin-type compounds; *Clin Pharmacokinet*, 39:255-270.

Nayyar P et al. (2012): Poor quality antimalaria drugs in Southeast Asia and Sub-Saharan Africa; *Lancet Infect Dis*, 12:488-490.

Nelsen TS, Schrecber SL (2008): Towards the optimal screening collection: A synthesis strategy; *Augew Chem Int Ed Engl*, 47:48-56.

Newton CRJ, Krishna S (1998): Severe falciparum malaria in children: current understanding of pathophysiology and supportive treatment; *Pharmacol Ther;* 79:1-53.

Newton PN et al. (2008): A collaborative epidemiological investigation into the criminal fake artesunate trade in South East Asia; *Plos Med*, 5:e32.

Newton P et al. (2011): Poor quality vital antimalarial in Africa: an urgent neglected public health priority; *Mal J*, 10:352.

Nieuwenhuis JA et al. (2006): Automated erythrocytapheresis in severe falciparum malaria: A critical appraisal; *Acta Trop*, 98:201-206.

Nilsen A, LaCrue AN, While KL, et al. (2013): Quinolones-3-diarylethers: a new class of antimalarial drugs; *Sci Transl Med*, 5:177ra37.

Noedl H, Walther H, et al. (2002): Histidine- rich protein II: A novel approach to malaria drug sensitivity testing; *Antimicrob Agents Chemother*, 46:1658-1664.

Nonaka D et al. (2012): Content Analysis of Primary and Secondary Scholl Textbooks regarding malaria control: A Multi-country Study; *Plos One*, 7:e36629.

Nosten F, ter Kuile FO, et al. (1991): Malaria during pregnancy in an area of unstable endemicity; *Trans R Soc Trop Med Hyg*; 85: 424-429.

Nosten F et al. (1993): Cardiac effects of antimalarial treatment with halofantrine; *Lancet*, 431:1054-1056.

Nosten F et al. (2000): Effects of artesunate-mefloquine combination on the incidence of Plasmodium falciparum malaria and mefloquine resistance in Western Thailand: a prospective study; *Lancet*, 356:297-302.

Nzila AM, Mberu EK, et al. (2002): Genetic diversity of Plasmodium falciparum parasites from Kenya is not affected by antifolate drug selection; *Int J Parasitol*, 32:1469-1476.

Nájera JA. *Malaria control: achievements, problems and strategies*. Geneva, WHO, 1999 (WHO/CDS/RBM/99.10) (*http://whqlibdoc.who.int/hq/1999 /WHO_MAL_99.1087.pdf*).

Narasimhan V, Attaran A (2003): Roll Back Malaria? The scarcity of international aid for malaria control. *Mal J*, 2:8.

Newton CRJ, et al. (1990): Cerebral malaria: what is unarousable coma? *Lancet*, 335:472;

Ngomane, L. & C. de Jager (2012): Changes in Malaria morbidity and mortality in Mpumalanga Province, South Africa (2001-2009): a retrospective study; *Malaria J*, 11:19.

Noedl, H., K.et al. (2006): Sensitivity and specificity of an antigen detection ELISA for malaria diagnosis. *Am. J. Trop. Med. Hyg*. 75:1205–1208.

Noedl H et al. (2008): Evidence of artemisinin resistant malaria in Western Cambodia; *NEJM*, 359:2619-2620.

Oduola AM et al. (2011): Plasmodium falciparum: evaluation of lactate dehydrogenase in monitoring therapeutic response to standard to antimalarial drugs in Nigeria; *Exp Parasitol*, 87:283-289.

Oliver SG (1996): From DNA sequence to biological function; *Nature*, 379:597-600.

Ollomo B, Durand P, Prugnolle F, et al. (2009): A new malaria agent in African hominids; PLoS Pathog, 5:e1000446. doi: *10.1371/journal. ppat.1000446.*

O'Meara WP et al. (2010): Change in the burden of malaria in Sub Saharan Africa; *Lancet*, 10:545-555.

Osafo-Addo AD et al. (2008): HLA-DRB1*04 allele is associated with severe malaria in Northern Ghana; *Am J Trop med Hyg*, 78:251-255.

OECD (2008): *The economic Impact of Counterfeit and piracy.*

Ogutu B, Tiono AB, et al. (2012): Treatment of asymptomatic carriers with artemether-lumefantrine: an opportunity to reduce the burden of malaria? *Mal J* 9:30

Ohrt C, Mirabelli-Primdahl L, et al. (1997) Distinguishing Plasmodium falciparum treatment failures from reinfection by restriction fragment length polymorphism and polymerase chain reaction genotyping. *American Journal of Tropical Medicine and Hygiene* 57, 430–437.

Ojo KK, Pfander C, et al. (2012): Transmission of malaria to mosquitoes blocked by bumped kinase inhibitors; *J Clin Inves*t, 122:2301-22035.

Oluwale, O., Sea S. & Mohammed M. (2010): Plasmodium falciparum-induced kidney and liver dysfunction in malaria patient in Free Town Sierra Leone; *SLJBR*, 2:70-74.

Oliveira TYK, Haris EE, et al. (2012): Molecular evolution of a malaria resistance gene (DARC) in primates; *Immunogenetics*, 64:497-505.

Olszewski KL, Llinas M (2013): Extraction of hydrophilic metabolites from Plasmodium falciparum-infected erythrocytes for metabolomics analysis; *Methods Mol Bio*, 923:259-266.

Olszewski K L et al. (2009): Host-parasite interactions revealed by Plasmodium falciparum metabolomics; *Cell Host Microbe* 5, 191–199.

Olszewski KL, Mather MW, et al. (2013): Retraction: Branched Tricarboxylic acid metabolism in *Plasmodium falciparum*; doi: 10.1038/nature12164.

Olutu AI et al. (2009): Further analysis of correlates of protection from a phase 2a trial of the falciparum malaria vaccine RTS, S/ASO1B and RTS, S/ASO2A in malaria-naïve adults; *J Infect Dis*, 201:970-971.

Olutu A et al. (2011): Efficacy of RTS, S/ASO1E malaria vaccine and exploratory analysis in anti-circumsporozoite antibody titres and protection in children aged 5-17 months in Kenya and Tanzania: a randomised controlled trial; *Lancet Infect Dis*, 11:102-109.

Ong'echa JM, Davenport GC, et al. (2011): *Identification of Inflammatory Biomarkers for Pediatric Malaria /Anemia Severity using Novel Statistical Methods*, doi:10.1128/IAI.05161-11.

Orjih AU (1996): Heamolysis of Plasmodium falciparum trophozoite-infected erythrocyte after artemisinin exposure; *Br J Haematol*, 92:324-328.

Oyelade J, et al. (2010): Computational identification of signaling pathway in Plasmodium falciparum; *Infect Genet Evol*, 11:755-764.

Panday AV, Bisht H, et al. (2001): Mechanisms of malaria haem detoxification inhibition of chloroquine; *Biochem J*, 355:333-338.

Papalexis V, Siomos M, et al. (2001): Histidine-rich protein 2 of the malaria parasite, Plasmodium falciparum is involved in detoxification of the by-products of heamoglobin degradation; *Mol Biochem Parasitol*, 115:77-86.

Parise ME, et al. (1998): Efficacy of sulphadoxine-pyrimethamine for prevention of placental malaria in an area of Kenya with a high prevalence of malaria and human immunodeficiency virus infection; *Am J Trop med Hyg*, 59:822.

Patz JA & RB Kovats (2005): Hotspots in climate change and human health; *BMJ*, 325:1049-1098.

Pigott DM et al. (2012): Funding for malaria control 2006-2010: A comprehensive global assessment; *Mal J*, 11:246.

Piper R. et al. (1999): Immunocapture diagnostic assays for malaria using plasma lactate dehydrogenase (pLDH); *Am J Trop med Hyg*, 60:109-118.

Pohlit AM, Lima RBS, Frausin G, et al. (2013): Amazonian plant natural products: perspective for discovery of new antimalarial drug leads; *Molecules*, 16:9219-10.

Pollack, Y.T. et al. (1982): The genome of *Plasmodium falciparum* I. DNA base composition; *Nucl. Acids Res*, 10:539–546

Pouville B, Buffet P. A., Lepolard C, et al. (2000): Cytoadhesin of Plasmodium falciparum ring-stage-infected erythrocytes. *Nat. Med.* 6:1264–126

Prugnolle F, et al. (2011): African monkeys are infected by *Plasmodium falciparum* nonhuman primate-specific strains; *Proc Natl Acad Sci USA*, 108: 11948–11953.

Pacheco MA, Cranfield M, et al. (2013): Malaria parasite diversity in chimpanzees: the value of comparative approaches to ascertain the evolution of Plasmodium falciparum; *Mal J*, 12:328.

Paget-McNicol, S et al. (2001): Mutation rates in the dihydrofolate reductase gene of Plasmodium falciparum; *Parasitology*, 122:497-505.

Parroche P et al. (2007): Malaria hemozoin is immunologically inert but radically enhances innate response by presenting malaria DNA to Toll-like receptor 9; *PNAS*, 104:1919-1924.

Pattanasin, S. et al. (2003): Evaluation of a new Plasmodium lactate dehydrogenase assay (OptiMal-IT) for the detection of malaria; *Trans R Soc Trop Med Hyg*; 97:672-674.

Patil S, Suryavanash S, et al. (2013): Evaluation of novel lipid based formulation of β-Artemether and Lumefantrine in murine malaria model; *Int J Pharma*, 455:229-234.

Paul REL, Brockman A, Price RN et al. (1999) Genetic analysis of Plasmodium falciparum infections on the north-western border of Thailand. *Transactions of the Royal Society of Tropical Medicine and Hygiene* 93, 587–593.

Pavithra SR, Kumar R, Tatu U (2007): Systems analysis of chaperone networks in the malarial parasite Plasmodium falciparum; *PLos Compul Biol*, 3:e168.

Pepe MS, Etzioni R, et al. (2001): Phases of biomarker development for early detection of cancer; *J Natl Cancer Inst*, 93:1054–1061.

Perimaan H et al. (1984): Antibodies in malarial sera to parasite antigen in the membrane of erythrocyte infected with early asexual stage; *J Exp Med*, 159:1686-1704.

Perrin LH et al. (1984): Immunization against Plasmodium falciparum asexual blood stage using soluble antigen; *Clin Exp Immunol*, 56:67-72.

Perrin LH et al. (1984): Antimalarial immunity in Saimiri monkeys; *J Exp Med*, 160:441-451.

Perry MJ et al. (2006): A prospective study of serum DDT and progesterone and estrogen levels across the menstrual cycle in nulliparious women of reproductive age; *Am J Epidemiol*, 104:1056-1064.

Phillips MA & PK Rathod (2010): Plasmodium dihydrorotate dehydrogenase: a primary target for novel anti-malarial chemotherapy; *Infect Disnd Drug Targets*, 10: 226-239.

Phillips R.S. (2001): Current Status of Malaria and Potential for Control, *Clin Microbiol Rev*, 14:208. DOI:10.1128/CMR.14.1.208-226.2001.

Picot S et al. (2009): A systematic review and meta-analysis of evidence for correlation between molecular markers of parasite resistance and treatment outcome in falciparum malaria; *Mal J*, 8:89.

Playford EG et al. (2002): Evaluation of the ICT malaria P.f/P.v. and the optimal rapid diagnostic tests for malaria in febrile returned travelers; *J Clin Microbiol*, 40:4166-4171.

Plouffe D et al. (2008): In silico activity profiling reveals the mechanism of action of antimalarial discovered in a high-throughput screen; *PNAS USA*, 105:9059-9064.

Pluess B et al. (2010): Indoor residual spraying for preventing malaria; *Cochrane Database Syst Rev,* 4: CD06657.

Pogo AO and Chaudhuri A (2000): The Duffy protein: a malarial and chemokine receptor. *Semin. Hematol*. 2:122-129.

Polley SD, Mori Y, Watson J, et al. (2010): Mitochondrial DNA targets increase sensitivity of malaria detection using loop-mediated isothermal amplification; *J Clin Microbiol*,48(8):2866-71.

Potocnjak P et al. (1980): Monovalent fragments (Fab) of monoclonal antibodies to sporozoites surface antigen; *J Exp Med*, 151:1504-1513.

Project for the accelerated implementation of malaria control in Africa (1997–1998). Geneva, RBM Partnership/WHO, 2000 (WHO/CDS/RBM/2000.27) http://whqlibdoc.who.int/hq/2000/WHO_CDS_RBM_2000.27.pdf).

Price RN, Nosten F et al. 1996. Effects of artemisinin derivative on malaria transmissibility; *Lancet*, 347:1654-1658.

Price RN, Douglas NM. 2009. Artemisinin combination therapy for malaria beyond good efficacy; *CID*, 49:1638-1640.

Purfield A et al. (2004): A new method for detection of pfmdr mutants in Plasmodium falciparum DNA doing real-time PCR; *Mal J*, 7:3-9.

Rabinowitz JD (2007): Cellular Metabolomics of *Escherichia coli*; *Expert Rev Proteomics*, 4:18-198.

Raghavendra K et al. (2011): Malaria vector controls: from past to future; *Parasitol Res*, 108: 757-779.

Ramharter M, et al. (2003): Cytokine profile of plasmodium- falciparum-specific T cells in non-immune malaria parasite; *Parasite Immunol*, 25:211-219.

Ramharter M et al. (2003): In vitro activity and interaction of clindamycin combined with dihydroartemisinin against Plasmodium falciparum; *Antimicrob Agents Chemother*; 47:3494-3499.

Ramharter M et al. (2005): Artesunate-clindamycin versus quinine-clindamycin in the treatment of plasmodium falciparum Malaria: a randomized controlled trials; *Clin Infect Dis*, 40:1777-1784.

Ramsdale CD & Hass E (1978): Some aspects of epidemiology of resurgent malaria in Turkey; *Trans Soc Trop Med Hyg*, 72:570-580.

Ranford-Cartwright LC, Taylor J. et al. (1997) Molecular analysis of recrudescent parasites in a Plasmodium falciparum drug efficacy trial in Gabon. *Transactions of the Royal Society of Tropical Medicine and Hygiene* 91, 719–724.

Ranford-Cartwright LC et al. (2002): Critical comparison of molecular genotyping methods for detection of drug resistance Plasmodium falciparum; *Trans R. Soc Trop Med Hyg*, 96:568-372.

Rao RU, et al. (2009): A qPCR based multiplex assay for the detection of *Wuchereria bancrofti*, Plasmodium falciparum and Plasmodium vivax DNA. *Trans. R. Soc. Trop. Med. Hyg.* 103, 365–370.

Rathod PK et al. (1997): Variation in frequencies of drug resistance in Plasmodium falciparum; *PNAS*, 94:9389-9393.

Raventos SC et al. (1985): Membrane knobs are required for the microcirculator obstruction induced by Plasmodium falciparum infected erythrocyte; *PNAS USA*, 82:3829-3833.

Ra RN, Chatterjea JB and Chaudhuri RN (1964): Observations on the resistance in HbE thalassemia disease to induced infection with Plasmodium vivax. *Bull. W. H. O.* 30:51-55.

Reaves ML, Rabinowitz JD (2011): Metabolomics in systems microbiology; *Current Opin Biotechnol*, 22:17-25

RBM (2005): *Global strategic plan: Roll Back Malaria 2005-2015* Geneva: Roll Back Malaria Partnership.

Repetto EC, Traverso A & Giacomazzi CG (2011): Possible clinical failure of arthemether-lumefantrine in an Italian traveler with uncomplicated falciparum malaria; *Meditrr JHematol Infect Dis*, 3:e2011041.

Reyburn, H et al. (2007): Rapid diagnostic tests compared with malaria microscopy for guiding outpatient treatment of febrile illness in Tanzania: randomised trial. *BMJ* 334:403.

Rich, S. M et al. (1998): Malaria's Eve: evidence of a recent population bottleneck throughout the world populations of Plasmodium falciparum. *Proc. Natl. Acad. Sci. USA* 95:4425-4430.

Richie TL & Saul A (2002): Progress and challenges for malaria vaccine; *Nature*, 415:694-701.

Riddle MS et al. (2002): Exchange transfusion on an adjunct therapy in severe Plasmodium falciparum malaria: a meta-analysis; *Clin Infect Dis*, 34:1192-1198.

Rivera N, Romero SE, et al. (2013): Blackwater fever like in murine malaria; *Parasitology Res*, 112:1021-1029.

Roche PCR: *www.molecular.roche.com/pcr/pages/default.aspx* (Accessed 28/10/2013).

Rodriques MM et al. (1991): CD8+ cytotoxic T cells clones derived against the *Plasmodium yoelii* circumsporozoite protein protect against malaria; *Int Immunol,* 3:579-585.

Rogier, G., Imberts P, et al. Epidemiological and clinical aspects of black water fever and children suffering frequent malaria attacks. *Trans R Soc Trop Med Hyg*, 97:193-7.

Rogers W et al. (1992): Characterization of the gene encoding sporozoites surface protein 2, a protective Plasmodium yoelii sporozoites antigen; *Mol Biochem Parasitol*, 53:45-52.

Roll Back Malaria Partnership (2011): *A decade of partnership and results*; Geneva World Health Organization.

Rolling T, Schmiedel S, et al. (2012): Post-treatment haemolysis in severe imported malaria after intravenous artesunate: case report of three patients with Hyperparasitaemia; *Malaria J*, 11:169.

Romero P et al. (1989): Cloned cytotoxic T cells recognizes an epitope in the circumsporozoite protein and protect against malaria; *Nature*, 341:323-325.

Rottmann M, et al. (2010): Spiroindolines, a potent compound class for the treatment of malaria; *Science*, 329:1175-1180

Rowe, JA, Shafi J, et al. (2002): Nonimmune IgM, but not IgG binds to the surface of Plasmodium falciparum-infected erythrocytes and correlates with rosetting and severe malaria; *Am J Trop med Hyg*, 66: 692–699.

Rubio JM, Benito A, Roche J et al. (1999) Semi-nested, multiplex polymerase chain reaction for detection of human malaria parasites and evidence of Plasmodium vivax infection in Equatorial Guinea. *American Journal of Tropical Medicine and Hygiene* 60, 183–187.

Russell S (2004): The economic burden of illness for household in developing countries: catastrophic or manageable? A review of studies focusing on malaria, tuberculosis and human immunodeficiency virus/acquired immunodeficiency syndrome, *Am J Trop med Hyg*, 71: (Suppl 2): 147-155.

Ruwende CS, et al. (1995): Natural selection of hemi- and heterozygotes for G6PD deficiency in Africa by resistance to severe malaria; *Nature*, 376:246-249.

RSC: *www.rsc.org* (Accessed 27/10/2013).

Saenz FE, Lacrue AN, et al. (2013): 4-1-Quinolones and 1, 2, 3-tetrahydroacridine-9 (10H)-ores prevent the transmission of Plasmodium falciparum to *Anopheles freeborni*; AAC September 30 (Epub ahead of print)

Sana TB, Gordon DB, et al. (2013): Global mass spectrometry-based metabolomics profiling of erythrocyte infected with Plasmodium falciparum; *Plos One*, 8:e60840.

Satimai, W et al. (2012): Artemisinin resistance containments project in Thailand. I: responses to mefloquine –artesunate combination therapy among falciparum malaria patients in provinces bordering Cambodia; *Mal J*, 11:300.

Saul A (1999): The role of variant surface antigen on malaria-infected red blood cells; *Parasitol Today*, 15:455-451.

Schellenberg D et al. (2001): Intermittent treatment for malaria and anemia control at the time of routine vaccination in Tanzanian infants: A randomised-control trial; *Lancet*, 357:1471-1477.

Scherf, A., et al. (2008): Antigenic variation in Plasmodium falciparum; *Ann Rev Microbiol*, 62:445-470.

Schofield CJ & White GB (1984): House design and domestic vectors of diseases; *Trans R Soc Trop Med Hyg*, 78:285-292.

Schultz LJ et al. (1994): The efficacy of antimalarial regimen containing sulphadoxine-pyrimethamine and/or chloroquine in preventing peripheral and placental Plasmodium falciparum infection among pregnant women in Malawi; *Am J Trop med Hyg*, 51:515-522.

Shah I et al. (1997): Chloroquine resistance in Pakistan and the upsurge of falciparum malaria in Pakistani and Afghan refugee population, *Am Trop Med Parasitol*, 91: 591-602.

Shankarkumar U (2004): The Human Leukocyte Antigen (HLA) System; Int. J *Hum Genet*, 4:91-103.

Shi C et al. (1990): Changes in weight gain and anemia attributable to malaria in Tanzanian children living under holoendemic condition; *Trans R Soc Trop Med & Hyg*, 90:262-265.

Shiff CT (1998): Vector control, community participation and malaria morbidity in the Bagamoyo district of Rural Tanzania; *Res Rev Parasitol*, 58:209-215.

Shkurti K, Vyshka G, et al. (2013): Imported malaria in Albania and the risk factors that could allow its reappearance; *Mal J*, 12:197.

Shulman CE et al. (1999): Intermittent sulphadoxine-pyrimethamine to prevent severe anemia secondary to malaria in pregnancy: A randomised placebo-controlled trial; *Lancet*, 352:632-636.

Sibley CH et al. (2001): Pyrimethamine-sulfadoxine resistance in Plasmodium falciparum: What next? *Trends Parasitol*, 17:582-588.

Siddique WA et al. (1987): Merozoite surface coat precursor protein completely protects Aotus monkeys against Plasmodium falciparum; *PNAS*, 84:3014-3018.

Sidhu AB et al. (2007): In vitro efficacy, resistance selection and structural modeling studies implicate the malaria parasite apicoplast as the target of azithromycin; *J Biol Chem*, 282: 2494-2504

Sim BKL et al. (1990): Primary structure of the 175K Plasmodium falciparum erythrocyte binding antigen and identification of a peptide which elicits antibodies that inhibit malaria merozoites invasion; *J Cell Biol*, 111:1877-1884.

Singh B, et al. (2004): A large focus of naturally acquired *Plasmodium knowlesi* infections in human beings. *Lancet* 363: 1017–1024.

Sipilanyambe N et al. (2008): From chloroquine to artesunate –lumefantrine: the process of drug policy change in Zambia; *Mal J*, 7:25.

Sirawaraporn, W. et al. (1997): Antifolate-resistant mutants of Plasmodium falciparum dihydrofolate reductase; *PNAS USA*, 94:1124-1129.

Smith JD, et al. (1995): Switches in expression of Plasmodium falciparum var genes correlate with changes in antigenic and cytoadherent phenotypes of infected erythrocytes; *Cell*, 82: 101–110.

Smith RC et al. (2012): Regulation of Anti-Plasmodium Immunity by a LITAF-like Transcription Factor in the Malaria vector *Anopheles gambiae*; *PLoS Pathogen*, 8:e1002965.

Smythe JA et al. (1988): Identification of 2 integral membrane protein of Plasmodium falciparum; *PNAS*, 85:5195-5199.

Snounou G, Pinheiro L, Goncalves A et al. (1993):The importance of sensitive detection of malaria parasites in the human and insect hosts in epidemiological studies, as shown by the analysis of field samples from Guinea Bissau. *Transactions of the Royal Society of Tropical Medicine and Hygiene* 87, 649–653.

Snounou G & Beck H-P (1998): The use of PCR genotyping in the assessment of recrudescence or reinfection after antimalarial treatment. *Parasitology Today* 14, 462–467.

Snow RW & K March (2010): Malaria in Africa: Progress and Prospect in the decade since Abuja Declaration; *Lancet*, 376:137-139.

Som MF et al. (2007): Economic burden of malaria in rural Tanzania: variation by socioeconomic status and season; *Trop Med & Int Health*, 12:1139-1147.

Stevenson M.M. et al. (1995): IL-12-induced protection against blood-stage Plasmodium chabaudi AS requires IFN-gamma and TNF-alpha and occurs via a nitric oxide-dependent mechanism; *Immunol J*, 155(5):2545–56.

Stoddard ST, et al. (2009): The role of human movements in the transmission of vector-borne pathogens; *PLoS Negl Trop DIs*, 3:e481.

St Sauver JL et al. (2002): Association between human leukocyte antigen homozygosity and antibody levels to measles vaccine; *J Infect Dis*, 185:1545-1549.

Su XZ et al. (1998): The large diverse gene family var encodes protein involved in Cytoadherence of Plasmodium falciparum-infected erythrocytes; *Cell*, 82:89-100.

Sun P et al. (2003): Protective immunity induced with malaria vaccine, RTS,S is linked to Plasmodium falciparum circumsporozoite protein-specific CD4+ and CD8+ T cell producing IFN-gamma; *J Immunol*, 171:6961-6967.

Suwanaruski R, Russell B, et al. (2007): Chloroquine resistant Plasmodium vivax: in vitro characterization and association with molecular polymorphism; *Plos One*, 2:e1089.

Szczopiokowski ZM et al. (2010): Guidelines on the use of therapeutic apheresis in clinical medicine, *Society for Apheresis J clin Apher*, 25:83-177.

Tako, E.A., A. Zhou, J. Lohoue, et al. (2005): Risk factors for placental malaria and its effect on pregnancy outcome in Yaoundé, Cameroon, *Am J Trop med Hyg*; 72:236-242.

Talisuna AO et al. (2012): The Affordable medicines facility-malaria-A success in peril; *Mal J*, 11:370.

Tan PL et al. (2001): Twin studies of immunogenicity-determining the genetic contribution to vaccine failure; *Vaccine*, 19:2434-2439.

Targett, G, Drakeley C, et al. (2001): Artesunate reduces but does not prevent post-treatment transmission of Plasmodium falciparum to Anopheles gambiae; *J Infect Dis*, 183:1254-1259.

Tatem AJ, Rogers DJ, Hay SI (2006): Global transport networks and infectious diseases spread; *Adv Parasitol*, 62:293-343.

Tatensky A et al. (2011): Preventing the Reintroduction of malaria in Mauritius: A programmatic and financial assessment; *Plos One*, 6: e23832.

Taudon N et al. (2008): Qualitative analysis of a bis-thiazolium antimalarial compounds SAR97276, in mouse plasma-red blood cell samples, using liquid chromatography mass spectrometry; *J Pharm Biomed Annal*, 46: 148-156.

Taylor TE, Wirima JJ, Molyneun ME, Davis TME, Brewster DR, Hill AVS, et al. (1990): Hypoglycaemia and cerebral malaria; *Lancet*, 336:950-1.

Taylor T. et al. (2006): Standardized data collection for multi-center clinical studies of severe malaria in African children: establishing the SMAC network; *Trans R Soc Trop Med Hyg*, 100(7):615–22.

Thanh NX, Trung TN, et al. (2012): The efficacy and tolerability of artemisinin-piperaquine (Artequick®) versus artesunate-amodiaquine (Coarsucam) for the treatment of uncomplicated Plasmodium falciparum malaria in south-central Vietnam; *Malaria J*, 11:217.

The RTS, S Clinical Trials Partnership (2011): First results of phase 3 trial of RTS, S/ASO1 malaria vaccine in African children; *NEJM*, 265: 1863-75.

Tishkoff SA, et al. (2001): Haplotype diversity and linkage disequilibrium at human G6PD: recent origin of alleles that confer malarial resistance; *Science*, 293:455-462.

Tjitra E, Hasugian AR, et al. (2012). Efficacy and safety of artemisinin-naphthoquine versus dihydroartemisinin-piperaquine in adult patients with uncomplicated malaria: a multi-centre study in Indonesia; *Malaria J*, 11:153.

Thibodeau SN (1994): Recent applications of PCR in Clinical Laboratory Medicine; *Clin Chem*, 40:681-682.

Tsuruta H et al. (2009): High-level production of amorpha-4,11-diene, a precursor of the antimalarial agent artemisinin in *Escherichia coli; Plos One*, 4: e4489.

Trape J-F et al. (1998): Impact of chloroquine resistance on malaria mortality; *C.R. Acad Sci Ser III*, 321:689-697.

Trape J-F, Tall A, et al. (2011): Malaria morbidity and pyrethroid resistance after introduction of insecticide-treated bednets and artemisinin-based combination therapies: a longitudinal study; *Lancet Infect Dis*, 11:925-932.

Tran TH, Day NP, et al. (1996): A controlled trial of arthemether or quinine in Vietnamese adults with severe falciparum malaria; *NEJM*, 335: 76-83.

Trant TT et al. (1992): Acute renal failure in patients with severe falciparum malaria; *Clin Infect Dis*, 24:564-569.

Tredger JM & Sherwood RA (1997): The liver: New functional, prognostic diagnostic tests; *Am Clin Biochem*, 34: 121-141.

Triglia T, Wang P, et al. (1998): Allelic exchange at the endogenous genomic locus in Plasmodium falciparum proves the role of dihydropteroate synthese in sulfadoxine-resistant malaria; *EMBO J*, 17:3807-15.

Tschan S, Brouwer AJ, et al. (2013): Broad-spectrum antimalarial activity of peptide sulfonyl fluorides: a new class of proteasome inhibitors, *AAC*, 57:3576-84.

Ramasamy R & SN Surendran (2011): Possible impact of rising sea levels on vector-borne infectious diseases; *BMC Infect Dis*, 11:18.

Ramasamy R & SN Surendra (2012): Global climate change and its potential impact on disease transmission by salinity-tolerant mosquito vector in coastal zones; *Frontiers in Physiology*, 3:198.

Reiter P (2008): Global warming and malaria: knowing the horse before the hitching the cart; *Mal J*, 7(Suppl 1):S3.

Roberts L, Enserink M (2007): Did they really say…eradication? *Science*, 318:1544–45.

Rock EP, Marsh K, et al. (1987): Comparative analysis of the *Plasmodium falciparum* histidine-rich proteins HRP1, HRP2 and HRP3 in malaria diagnosis of diverse origin; *Parasitology*, 95:209–227.

Report of the second African Malaria Conference. Geneva, WHO, 1956 (WHO/MAL/160, Lagos Conf. /32) (*http://whqlibdoc.who.int/malaria/WHO_Mal_160.pdf*).

Rudin W, Eugster HP, et al. (1997): Resistance to cerebral malaria in tumor necrosis factor- alpha /beta-deficient mice is associated with a reduction of intercellular adhesion molecule-1 up-regulation and T helper type 1 response; *Am. J. Pathol*, 150:257–266.

Rulisa S, Kaligirwa N, et al. (2012): Pharmacovigilance of arthemether-lumefantrine in pregnant women followed until delivery in Rwanda; *Malaria J*, 11:225.

Saito-Ito A., Y. Akai, S. He, M. Kimura, and M. Kawabata (2001): A rapid simple and sensitive flow cytometric system for detection of *Plasmodium falciparum; Parasitol. Int.* 50:249–257.

Seth AK, Nijhawan VS, et al. (1997): Malarial hepatic incidence and liver morphology; *Indian J of Gastroent*., 16 (Supplement 2): A107.

Slater AF (1996): Chloroquine: Mechanism of drug action and resistance in *Plasmodium falciparum*; *Pharmacol Ther*, 57:203-235.

Spielman A, et al. (1988): Malaria diagnosis by direct observation of centrifuged samples of blood. *Am. J. Trop. Med. Hyg*. 39:337–342.

Shiff CJ, et al. (1993): The rapid manual Para- Sight-F test. A new diagnostic tool for Plasmodium falciparum infection; *Trans. R. Soc. Trop. Med. Hyg*, 87:646–648.

Steketee RW, et al. (1996): Impairment of a pregnant woman's acquired ability to limit Plasmodium falciparum by infection with human immunodeficiency virus type-1; *Am J Trop med Hyg*, 1996; 55:49.

Sutherst RW (2004): Global change and humans vulnerability to vector-borne diseases; *CMR*, 17:136-173.

Sumbele IUN, Samje M, Nkuo-Akamji T (2013): A longitudinal study on aneamia in children with Plasmodium falciparum infection in the Mount Camerron region: prevalence, risk factors and perceptions by caregivers; *BMC Infect Dis*, 13:123.

Swarthout, TD et al. (2007): Paracheck-pf accuracy and recently treated Plasmodium falciparum infection: is there rick of over-diagnosis? *Mal J*, 6:58.

Tarimo DL et al. (2012): Malaria diagnosis and treatment under the strategy of the integrated management of childhood illness (IMCI): relevance of laboratory supports from the rapid immunochromatographic tests of ICT malaria P.f/p.v and Optimal; *Am Trop Med Parasitol*, 95:437-447.

ter Kuile FO, Parise ME, Verhoeff FH, Udhayakumar V, Newman RD (2004):The burden of co-infection with human immunodeficiency virus type 1 and malaria in pregnant women in sub-saharan Africa; *Am J Trop med Hyg*,71:54.

Turner G. D. H., Morrison H., Jones M., Davis T. M. E (1994): An immunohistochemical study of the pathology of fatal malaria—evidence for widespread endothelial activation and a potential role for intercellular adhesion molecule-1 in cerebral sequestration. *Am. J. Pathol.* 145:1057–1069.

Udomsangpetch R, et al. (1995): Rosette formation by Plasmodium vivax. *Trans R Soc Trop Med Hyg*; 89: 635-637.

Uhlemann AC et al. (2005): Amplification of plasmodium falciparum multidrug resistance gene 1 in isolates from Gabon; *J Infect Dis*, 192:1830-1835.

UNAIDS/WHO (2007) Ethical considerations in biomedical HIV prevention trials: UNAIDS/WHO guidance document on *http://data.unaids.org /pub/manual/2007/jci349_ethics_2_11_07en.pdf* (Accessed on 02/11/2012).

United Nations: United Nations Millennium Development New York: United Nations *http://www.un.org/millennium/declaration/ares552e.htm*.

Use of Malaria Rapid Diagnostic Tests on *http://searo.who.int/LinkFiles/ Malaria_in_the_SEAR_RDTGUIDELINES_final.pdf* (Access 30/11/2012).

Uzeugbu U.E. & Emeka CB (2011): Changes in liver function biomarkers among malaria infected patients in Ikeja Lagos State Nigeria; *Curr Research J Biol Sci,* 3:172-174.

Vachon F et al. 1990: Treatment of severe malaria by exchange transfusion; *NEJM*, 322:58-59.

Valea I. et al. (2009): Performance of OptiMAL-IT compared to microscopy for malaria detection in Burkina Faso; *Trop Med Int Health*, 14:338-340.

Valecha N et al. (2010): Arterolane, a new synthetic trioxolane for treatment of uncomplicated Plasmodium malaria: a phase II, multicenter, randomized dose-finding clinical trials; *Clin Infect Dis*, 51:684-691.

Van den Eede, P., V.E. Soto-Calle, et al. (2011): Plasmodium Vivax Sub-Patent Infection after Radical Treatment Are Common in Peruvian Patients: Results of 1-Year Prospective Cohort Study; *PLOS ONE*, 6: e16257.

Van Genderen JJP et al. (2012): Trends in the knowledge, attitudes and practices of travel risk groups towards prevention of malaria: results from the Dutch Schipol Airport Survey 2002 to 2009; *Mal J*, 11:79.

Vanloubbeeck Y, Pickyangkul S, et al. (2013): Comparison of the immune responses induced by soluble and particulate Plasmodium viva circumsporozoite vaccine candidate formulated in ASO1 in rhesus macaques; Vaccine, *doi.10.1016/j.vaccine.2013.10.041* (Epub ahead of print)

Verhoeff FH et al. (1998): An evaluation of the effects of intermittent sulfadoxine-pyrimethamine treatment in pregnancy on parasite clearance and risk of low birth weight in rural Malawi; *Am Trop Med Parasitol*, 92:141-150.

Vermenleu AN et al. (1985): Sequential expression of antigen in asexual stage of Plasmodium falciparum accessible to transmission-blocking antigen antibodies in mosquito; *J Exp Med*, 162:1460-1476.

Versiani FG, Almeida ME, et al. (2013): N-terminal Plasmodium vivax merozoites surface protein-1, a potential subunit for malaria vivax vaccine; Clinical & Dev Immunology, *doi.org/10.1155/2013/965841.*

Venners SA et al. (2005): Preconception serum DDT and pregnancy loss: a prospective study using a biomarker of pregnancies; *Am J Epidemiol*, 162:709-716.

Viroj W (2006): Co-infection between tuberculosis and malaria: a consideration on interaction of molecules and pathogenesis; *J Vect Borne Dis*, 43:195-197.

Vivas L et al. (2007): Antimalarial efficacy and drug interaction of the novel semi-synthetic endoperoxide artemisome in vitro and in vivo; *J Antimicrob Chemother*, 59:658-665.

Warrell DA et al. (1982): Dexamethasone proves deleterious in cerebral malaria, A double blind trial in 100 comatose patients; *NEJM*, 306:313-319.

Watanabe J, M. Suzuki, et al. (2001): FULL- malaria: a database for full-length enriched cDNA library from human malaria parasite, *Plasmodium falciparum; Nucleic Acids Res*, 29:70-71.

Watanabooyong P et al. (2011): Rapid increase in parasitaemia following red cell exchange for malaria; *J Clin Apher*, 26:315-319.

Water A.P., D.G. Higgins, T.F. McCutchan (1991): Plasmodium falciparum appears to have arisen as a result of lateral transfer between avian and human hosts; *PNAS*, 88:3140-3144.

Water AP, Higgins DG, McCutchan TF (1993): Evolutionary relatedness of some primate models of Plasmodium; *Mol Biol Evol*, 10:914-923.

Watkins WM and M Mosabo (1993): Treatment of Plasmodium falciparum malaria with pyrimethamine-sulfadoxine selective pressure for resistance is a function of long elimination half-life; *Trans R Soc Trop Med Hyg*, 87:75-78.

Watkins WM et al. (1997): The efficacy of antifolate antimalarial combination in Africa: A predictive model based on pharmacodynamic and pharmacokinetic analyses; *Parasitol Today*, 13:459-464.

Weatherall D. J., and J. B. Clegg (2001): Inherited haemoglobin disorders: an increasing global health problem; *Bull WHO*, 79:704-712.

Weber J.L. (1988) Molecular biology of malaria parasites. *Exp. Parasitol.* 66, 143–170.

Webster J et al. (2005): *Protecting all pregnant women and children under five years, living in malaria endemic areas in Africa with insecticide treated mosquito nets,* Geneva Roll Back Malaria.

Wegmann TG, Lin H, Guilbert LJ, Mosmann TR (1993): Bidirectional cytokine interactions in the maternal-fetal relationship: is successful pregnancy a Th2 phenomenon? *Immunol Today*; 14: 353-356.

Weir EG et al. (2000): Automated RBC exchange for cerebral malaria; *Transfusion*, 40:702-7.

Weiss WR et al. (1992): A T-cell clone directed at the circumsporozoite protein which protects mice against both Plasmodium yeolii and Plasmodium berghei; *J Immunol*, 149:2103-2109.

Wells TN et al. (2010): New medicines to improve control and contribute to eradication of malaria; *Nat Rev Drug Discover*, 8:879-891.

Wellems JR and Taylor DW (1986): Secretion of a malarial histidine- rich protein (Pf HRP II) from Plasmodium falciparum-infected erythrocytes; *J. Cell Biol*, 103:1269–1277.

Were T. et al. (2006): Suppression of RANTES in children with Plasmodium falciparum malaria; *Haematologica*, 91(10):1396–9.

West PA, Protopopoff N, et al. (2013): Malaria risk factors in North west Tanzania: the effects of spraying, nets and wealth; *Plos One*, 8:e65787.

Whalin B et al. (1984): Human antibodies to a Mr 155,000 Plasmodium falciparum antigen efficiently inhibit Merozoite invasion; *PNAS*, 81: 7912-7916.

White NJ, Nosten F, Looareesuwan S, et al. (1999): Averting a malaria disaster; *Lancet*, 353:1965–67.

White NJ (1996): The treatment of malaria; *NEJM*, 335:800-6.

White NJ (1999): Antimalarial drug resistance and combination chemotherapy; *Philos Trans R Soc London B. Biol Sci*; 354:739-741.

White NJ (2002): The assessment of antimalaria drug efficacy; *Trends Parasitol*, 18:458-464.

White NJ & W Pongtavornpinyo (2003): The de novo selection of drug resistance malaria parasites; *Proc Biol Sci*, 270:545-554.

White NJ et al. (2010): The murine cerebral malaria phenomenon; *Trends Parasitol*, 26:11-15.

White VA, Lewallen S, Beare N, Kayira K, Carr RA, Taylor TE (2001): Correlation of retinal haemorrhages with brain haemorrhages in children dying of cerebral malaria in Malawi; *Trans R Soc Trop Med Hyg*, 95:618-621.

White TEK, et al. (2006): Artesunate-induced depletion of embryonic erythroblasts preceded embryo lethality and teratogenicity in vivo; *Birth Defects Res*, 77:413-429.

Wiesner J et al. (2003): Fomidomycin for the treatment of malaria; *Parasitol Res*, 90: Suppl 2): S71-S76.

Windham GC et al. (2005): Exposure to organochlorine compounds and effects on ovarian function; *Epidemiology*, 16; 182-190.

Win TT, Jalloh A, et al. (2004): Molecular analysis of *Plasmodium ovale* variants. *Emerg. Infect. Dis*. 10:1235–1240.

Winskill P, Rowland M, et al. (2012): Malaria risk factor in north—east Tanzania; *Mal J*, 10:98.

Winstanley PA et al. (1992): The deposition of oral and intramuscular pyrimethamine-sulfadoxine in Kenyan children with high parasitaemia but clinically non-severe falciparum malaria; *Br J Clin Pharmacol*, 33:143-148.

Winstanley PA et al. (1993): Towards optimal parenteral quinine regimens for young children with malaria: importance of unbound quinine concentration; *Trans R Soc Trop Med Hyg*, 87:201-206.

Witt R, et al. (2010): Neopterin and Procalcitonin are suitable biomarkers for exclusion of severe Plasmodium Falciparum disease at the initial clinical assessment of travellers with imported malaria; *Malaria J*, 9:255.

Wongsrichanalai C & SR Meshnick (2008): Declining artesunate-mefloquine efficacy against falciparum malaria on the Cambodian-Thailand border; *Emerg Infect Dis*, 14:716-719.

Wong RPM et al. (2012): In vitro antimalaria activity and drug interaction of fenofibric acid; *Antimicrob Agents Chemother*, 56: 2814-2818.

Woodrow CJ et al. (2005): Artemisinins; *Postgrad Med J*, 81:71-78.

World Bank (2005): *Up to $500million more available for fight against malaria in Africa.*

World Health Organization (1951): *Report of the Malaria Conference in Equatorial Africa.* Geneva, World Health Organization.

World Health Organization Interim Commission. *Expert Committee on Malaria - report on the first session.* Geneva, WHO, 1947 (*WHO.IC/79; WHO.IC/ Mal./4) (http:// whqlibdoc.who.int/malaria/WHO_IC_MAL_4.pdf*).

World Health Organization (2000): WHO/MAL/2000.1091. *New perspectives in malaria diagnosis.* World Health Organization, Geneva, Switzerland

World Health Organization (2000): Severe falciparum malaria, *Trans R. Soc Trop Med*; 94:1-90.

World Health Organization. The Abuja Declaration and the Plan of Action. [Accessed August 1, 2012]. Apr 252000.An extract from the African Summit on Roll Back Malaria, Abuja (*WHO/CDS/RBM/2000.17). http://www. rollbackmalaria.org/docs/abuja_declaration_final.htm*

World Health Organization (2000): Severe falciparum malaria; *Trans R Soc Trop Med Hyg* 2000, 94:S1-90; PMID: 11103309

World Health Organization (2000): Severe falciparum malaria; World Health Organization, Communicable Diseases Cluster; *Transactions of the Royal Society of Tropical Medicine and Hygiene*, 94(Suppl 1):S1–90.

World Health Organization (2006): *Vector control and personal protection*; Geneva World Health Organization.

World Health Organization (2007): *Malaria elimination: a field manual for low and moderate endemic countries*. Geneva: World Health Organization.

World Health Organization. World malaria report 2009 *http://www.who.int/malaria/world_malaria_report_2009/en/index.html* ([Accessed August 1, 2012].)

World Health Organization: Guidelines for the treatment of malaria. *WHO/HTM/MAL/20061108 ISBN 978 92 4 154694 2 2006:266.*

World Health Organization: *Turkmenistan certified malaria-free*, Geneva: World Health Organization *http://www.who.int/malaria/elimination/turkmenistan certifiedmalariafree/en/index.html* (Accessed on 10/09/2013).

World Health Organization (2010): Morocco certified malaria-free; *Wkly Epidemiol Rec*, 85:235-236.

World Health Organization [Internet]. *Guidelines for the treatment of malaria.* 2nd ed. 2010.

World Health Organization (2010): *World Malaria Report 2010* Geneva, Switzerland.

World Health Organization (2010): *Guideline for the treatment of malaria*; 2nd edition, Geneva WHO.

World Health Organization (2010): *Global report on antimalarial drug efficacy and drug resistance: 2000-2010*, Geneva Switzerland.

World Health Organization: World Malaria Report 2011 on *http:// factsheet/fs094/en/index.html* (Accessed on 02/11/2012).

World Health Organization (2010): *Guidance for the treatment of malarial; 2nd edition*. Geneva WHO.

World Health Organization (2011): *DDT in indoor residual spraying: human health aspects*; Geneva World Health Research Organization.

World Health Organization (2011): *World malaria report. Global malaria programme*. Gene: World Health Organization publication.

World Health Organization (2012): *World Malaria Report 2012*; Geneva Switzerland.

Wuchty S, Adams JH, et al. (2009): A comprehensive *Plasmodium falciparum* protein interaction map reveals a distinct architecture of core interactome; *Proteomics*, 9:1841-1849.

Yazdani SS, et al. (2004): Evaluation of immune responses elicited in mice against a recombinant malaria vaccine based on Plasmodium vivax Duffy binding protein; *Vaccine*, 22:3727-37.

Yoshida N et al. (1980): Hybridoma produces protective antibodies directed against the sporozoite stage of malaria parasite; *Science*, 207:71-73.

Yukich JO, Taylor C, et al. (2013): Travel history and malaria infection risk in a low-transmission setting in Ethiopia: a case control study; *Mal J*, 12:33.

Zell R (2004): Global climate change and the emergence/re-emergence of infectious diseases; *Arch J. Med Microb*, 293:16-26.

Zimmerman PA, et al. (1999): Emergence of FY*A (null) in a Plasmodium vivax-endemic region of Papua New Guinea. *Proc. Natl. Acad. Sci. USA* 96:1397.

About this Book

This book: It is a journey through the world of malaria with a discussion of issues relating to malaria.

The book is made up of six major chapters:

- History and classification
- Malaria parasite and its life cycle
- Recent advances in epidemiology of human malaria
- Pathogenesis and clinical features, update in malaria treatment
- Update in antimalaria treatment & resistance
- Malaria control strategies

The book discusses some powerful new techniques which are now advancing the field of malariology. The key features of the book are that it is written in simple English and based on a strong element of review in which original articles were analyzed. The journey through the world of malaria will be of great interest to parasitologists, biologists, healthcare professionals and policy makers who are interested in formulating policies that will optimize malaria control strategies.

About the Author

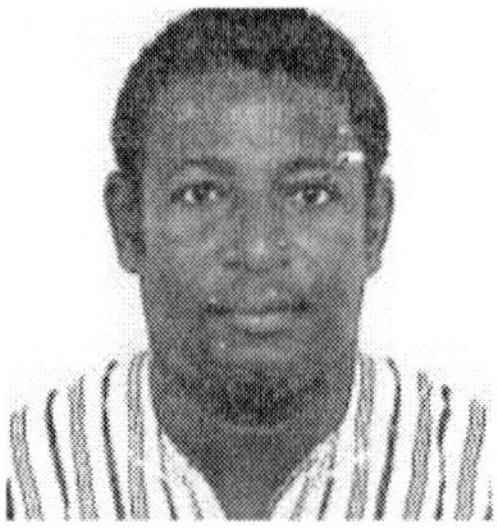

Abubakar Yaro is an Infectious Diseases Specialist. He is the Founder and CEO of Africa Health Research Organization, a non-profit making institution whose mission is promoting the reduction of disease burden and human suffering in Africa through evidence-based research, training and community-based intervention. He is also the Editor In Chief of Annals of Tropical Medicine & Public Health, the official publication of the organization. He is the CEO and President of Vis Viva Pharma Ltd, a R&D as well as distributor of pharmaceutical and personal care products. He is Founding Director and member of the Board of Trustees of Muslim Health Awareness Foundation

Publications by the same author:

- No Easy Route to Genuine Success.
- Ebola Fever Virus: A Natural Killing Machine.
- Essential Cervical Cancer
- Man, the wonderful creation of God
- Emerging Public Health Problems in Africa
- Near Death Experience: Facts or Fiction?

Index

B

D

E

H

I

J

K

N

O

P

Q

R

S

T

Y

Z